THE HOMOEOF
TREATMEN
SMALL ANIM
Principles & Practice

The Homoeopathic Treatment of Small Animals

Principles & Practice

CHRISTOPHER DAY
MA, VetMB, VetFFHom, MRCVS

RIDER
LONDON • SYDNEY • AUCKLAND • JOHANNESBURG

First published in Great Britain
by The C. W. Daniel Company Limited.
Reprinted 1990, revised edition 1992, reprinted 1996,
Revised and expanded 1998, reprinted 2004.
This edition published in 2005 by Rider,
an imprint of Ebury Publishing, Random House,
20 Vauxhall Bridge Road, London SW1V 2SA

www.randomhouse.co.uk

Addresses for companies within
The Random House Group Limited can be found at:
www.randomhouse.co.uk/offices.htm

The Random House Group Limited Reg. No. 954009

A CIP catalogue record for this book is available from the British Library

ISBN 9781844132898

This book gives non-specific, general advice and should not be relied on
as a substitute for proper veterinary or medical consultation. The author and
publisher cannot accept responsibility for illness arising out of the failure to
seek medical advice from a veterinarian.

The Random House Group Limited supports The Forest Stewardship
Council® (FSC®), the leading international forest-certification organisation.
Our books carrying the FSC label are printed on FSC®-certified paper.
FSC is the only forest-certification scheme supported by the leading
environmental organisations, including Greenpeace. Our
paper procurement policy can be found at
www.randomhouse.co.uk/environment

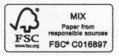

Printed and bound in Great Britain by Clays Ltd, St Ives plc

To Shelagh, my wife.
Her love, encouragement and untiring help
have been so valuable

To Carina, my baby daughter too,
who has proved to be such an inspiration

'. . . *In spite of this my pride does not prevent me from confessing that
veterinary surgeons . . . have more skill in the treatments of old wounds
than the most learned professors and members of the academics.*'

HAHNEMANN 1784

'*Peruvian (Cinchona) bark, which is used as a remedy for intermittent
fever, acts because it can produce symptoms similar to those of intermittent fever in healthy people.*'

HAHNEMANN 1790

Contents

Contents

Contents

Contents

Acknowledgements

This book is the result of a great deal of inspiration and education received from many directions. Firstly, my parents, who are both vets, have given me so much clinical guidance down the years. My mother, too has helped me to study homoeopathy. Much of her work in this field has inspired me to use the method myself and my uncle Bernhard, a homoeopathic doctor in Germany, has been a source of inspiration to me from an early age. The courses at the Faculty of Homoeopathy have been invaluable.

I would also like to thank Jørgen and Kirsten for their philosophical stimulation, Anthony for his helpful criticism, Trevor for his advice and encouragement, Christine, Sylvia and Thérèse and their animals for help in photography and, for her stoical efforts with the manuscript, my wife, Shelagh.

2nd Edition: Contributing to the modifications and additions in the 2nd Edition are the many patients and veterinary contacts that it has been my pleasure and honour to know in the intervening years.

3rd Edition: It is heartwarming that a third edition of the book is needed so soon. It is hoped that the book has been of value to the animals it is intended to serve and that their human companions are able to derive an understanding of homoeopathy which will enable a lifetime of development in this fascinating form of medicine. In the intervening years, so many animals and people have served to broaden and deepen my comprehension of homoeopathy and other therapies. I hope I am able to do justice to this development and to incorporate some of these advances in understanding in this new and widely

{xi}

reworked edition. My thanks go to Caroline Beaney for knocking much of my updated text into shape and to my publishers for their patience and help.

Preface

This book is planned as an introductory work on homoeopathy for use by both veterinarians and those who have animals and wish to try to help them at home. This has been a difficult compromise but very necessary on account of the wide demand for homoeopathy and the gross shortage of veterinary surgeons practising this form of medicine. Some sections will therefore take the subject too far for home treatment and others will necessarily appear too obvious to veterinarians. It is expected that veterinarians well-versed in the use of homoeopathy will want a more detailed reference section than this book contains but those in the early days of homoeopathic treatment will find it, I hope, an easy work of reference and a source of encouragement. Pet carers should be able to glean from its pages a wealth of easy to use remedies for common ailments in their pets and it should help them to understand the workings of homoeopathy, when a veterinarian's help should be sought and how best to help the vet to help the patient, by close observation of the symptoms.

A glance at the list of contents will show how the book is laid out, the brief notes in the list helping one to use the book for reference. Some sections will be especially of relevance to veterinarians and this will be obvious in the text. The book leaves out all reference to farm animals.

The 2nd and 3rd Editions carry an expanded index, in order to enhance the book's reference value, and a greater degree of cross-referencing appears in the text for the same purpose. The development of ideas since the 1st and 2nd Editions has produced some modifications and additions to the text. It is hoped that the reader will benefit from these changes and additions, which have incorporated some of the results of experience gained in the intervening years.

Introduction

The publication of this book is set amid an atmosphere of change in the thinking man's attitude to medicine, agriculture, diet, industry and environment.

The industrial revolution, the birth of modern medical ideas and the new agriculture, all of the late eighteenth century together with the accelerated loss and destruction of the natural environment and the appearance of 'easy foods' of the twentieth century have all grown hand in hand with population growth and social change. They have allowed redistribution of wealth, longer life, recession of the classical killer diseases, vast food production capacity and liberation of the housewife for career or recreation. The environment has suffered as population, travel and industry have grown. Nowadays, towards the end of the twentieth century, there is a growing awareness of the consequences of these trends. We are looking more and more into old and new ways of by-passing the harmful side of these changes, that is: shrinking of the natural environment, industrial pollution, widespread use of agricultural sprays and fertilisers, dietary impurities and drug side-effects. It would be quite wrong, however, to swing entirely in the opposite direction to these trends, running into danger of throwing the baby out with the bath water. It would not be right to react so wholeheartedly to these modern trends that we lose all advances. We must try to find the middle road where all that modern science has given us for the good of mankind can be retained and pick the best of what are either old or newly found methods in agriculture and horticulture, medicine, diet and health to keep us sound in mind and body.

For this reason one must wholeheartedly applaud efforts to make organic methods of farming more productive and profitable, efforts to research into the validity and mechanisms of natural medicines and efforts to eliminate from our diet processes, ingredients and additives which are harmful. We must examine very carefully the growing trend of genetic engineering and biotechnology and question the validity, wisdom, safety and ethics of such a path of development. Commercialism in all these fields must not be allowed to triumph over common sense and wisdom.

There is growing public interest in these fields which must be encouraged since demand usually promotes supply and this gradual shedding of public apathy, this awakening of a desire for more careful management by the powers-that-be, can only, in the long run, produce a more healthy and thoughtful approach by those that are involved in scientific advances. Science should take on more philosophy. There should be no war between the ideologies of natural medicine and conventional medicine, be it in the veterinary or human field. There should be mutual understanding and cross-pollination of ideas, leading to a new enlightenment and real advance in the philosophy and practice of medicine. It is for these reasons that I have tried, in this book, to draw attention to the scope of one form of natural medicine, homoeopathy, which I have studied and used for many years. Because I use several different natural therapies in an integrated programme I have almost no need for conventional drug medicine. I do however still, on very rare occasions, use conventional veterinary medicine when I feel it necessary so to do, therefore I do not intend this book to be a condemnation of conventional medicine but, rather, an illustration of ways in which natural medicine can help the health of pets without unnecessary use of chemicals and drugs. There seems to be a regrettable trend in orthodox medicine to believe that such drugs as antibiotics and corticosteroids can control most problems. If this were really so, why are more and more new and 'better' antibiotics needed? Antibiotics have their place but it is not the very prominent place they are given at present, by many today (see page 23).

In the first chapter explaining homoeopathy I have given many good reasons for using homoeopathy in place of conventional veterinary medicine. In some cases, conventional veterinary medicine can appear to achieve an equally good result and should not be totally dismissed. The reasons for use of this one (homoeopathic) system as opposed to another are not always an argument about which is the most effective method but a look into logic, the benefits and limitations of one method in a defined set of circumstances. I have attempted an objective assessment of principles; which approach led me to change to homoeopathy in the first place!

In the following chapters, I have tried to show the role of the veterinarian, the pet carer and the animal itself in achieving a cure.

Although this book is a handy reference book it should be studied carefully throughout, since many underlying principles of homoeopathic medicine are discussed in its pages. Use of the book only as a reference work defeats the philosophy of homoeopathy, in that this system of medicine is not used to treat diseases as such, but rather the patient itself, according to its individual response to disease, i.e. according to the totality of symptoms displayed. To look up, for instance, vomiting and its treatments in Chapter 8 and to use that remedy which seems immediately most obvious could fail to effect a cure, as a result of failure to take the whole patient into account. It is in this field that trained veterinarians can be essential to avoid needless suffering from protracted disease through wrong choices of remedy. By and large the chapter on veterinary involvement should act as a guide to where and when veterinary help is necessary.

What is probably most confusing at first, to those embarking on a study of homoeopathy, is the terminology and the naming of the remedies. These latter are listed at the end of the book with their common names. They are obtainable from various sources as described in Chapter 3 and should be carefully looked after according to a simple set of rules laid out in Chapter 7. A glossary can be found in the Appendix section to elucidate the more specialised terminology used in this book (and others).

A chapter of selected case histories is included in order to illustrate various points in the text and this should be read with a critical mind. Much can be learnt from the successes and failures of others.

Since the first edition of this book there have been many changes in attitudes to homoeopathy. The BMA published a report on 'alternative' medicine which showed a remarkable lack of objectivity by a body supposedly guided by objective principles. This body has since taken a much more enlightened and realistic view and, with the advent of more autonomy at local practice level, much more natural medicine is on offer to human patients, even under the NHS. The British Veterinary Association however, has sadly lagged far behind this forward-looking approach and, as yet, refuses to recognise the validity of veterinary homoeopathy of the BAHVS and of the Faculty of Homoeopathy qualification (at the time of writing). The media have given homoeopathy and other natural therapies tremendous exposure, not least in the veterinary field. The public appear to be more and more aware of, interested in and looking for natural therapies. The EC has outlawed growth promotion implants in beef and is addressing the problems of drug control on the farm. Farmers are taking to homoeopathy more than ever before. Veterinarians are able to take official courses, accredited by the Faculty of Homoeopathy, specially designed for them and leading to a qualification (*VetMFHom*, the first of its kind in the world). The International Association for Veterinary Homoeopathy was formed in Luxembourg in 1986 and serves as an unprecedented medium for the global exchange of veterinary homoeopathic knowledge, skills and understanding, not least through the pages of its International Journal for Veterinary Homoeopathy. Clinical research is making new strides, serving to further the understanding and acceptance of homoeopathic principles. Membership of the British Association of Homoeopathic Veterinary Surgeons has more than trebled in the intervening years. I believe a new era of understanding is in the making.

CHAPTER I

The Nature of Homoeopathy

All 'alternative' medicine practices tend to be lumped together in people's minds and homoeopathy is no exception. It is often confused with herbalism, faith healing, 'black box' medicine, radiaesthesia etc., which is not correct although perhaps some of them are related. All have a part to play but confusion of the systems serves no purpose. Homoeopathy is in reality one of the most scientific and precise forms of medicine available. This remark may seem difficult to justify but I hope to do so in this chapter. The following chapters should serve to illustrate the point.

Samuel Hahnemann in the late eighteenth century gave us formalised homoeopathy but the principle involved has been popping up in medical philosophy since Classical Greek times. Sadly it was never developed as a theory until Samuel Hahnemann's work, by which time new lines of scientific medicine were being explored. This chronology had repercussions on the later acceptability of homoeopathy. Up until this period medicine had been a very illogical hit and miss affair. It seemed that the more distasteful, pungent or unusual a medicine and the more dangerous, heroic or repulsive a technique, the more effective it was expected to be. There appeared to be little regard for negative results and what cures did occur most probably occurred as a result of the patient's inner strength triumphing over both the disease and the 'cure'.

DISCOVERY: LIKE CURES LIKE

Hahnemann became more and more disillusioned with medicine and devoted a greater proportion of his time and thought to his scholarly

{1}

work of translating medical texts into German, this despite his renown and prominence in the medical world. It was while translating the Materia Medica by William Cullen, a Scottish physician, that he embarked upon his adventure of discovery of homoeopathy. He disagreed with Cullen's explanation of the action of Cinchona bark against malaria, one of the few effective treatments of those days. In trying to find out the true mechanism he tested the drug on himself, producing symptoms indistinguishable from malaria in response!

He added a footnote to his translation of Cullen's Materia Medica questioning the proposed 'tonic' effect on the stomach as follows (I have updated the language):

'By combining the strongest bitters and the strongest astringents we can obtain a compound which, in small doses, possesses a more powerful tonic effect on the stomach than Cinchona bark, and yet no fever specific can be made from such a compound. The undiscovered principle of the effect of Cinchona bark is not easy to find. I took, for several days as an experiment, four drams of China (Cinchona), twice daily. My feet and fingertips etc., at first became cold. I became languid and drowsy and then my heart began to palpitate; my pulse became quick and hard, and an intolerable anxiety, trembling, prostration in all the limbs, pulsation in the head, redness of cheeks, thirst, (the symptoms usually associated with intermittent fever – Malaria) all made their appearance. These symptoms lasted from two to three hours every time and recurred only when I repeated the dose. I discontinued the medicine and I was once more in good health.'

This set his mind on the track of 'let like be cured by like' or *'similia similibus curentur'*. Hahnemann writes of his newly discovered Natural Law:

'Every medicine which, among the symptoms it can cause in a healthy body, reproduces those most present in a given disease, is capable of curing the disease in the swiftest, most thorough and most enduring fashion.'

Being a true scientist, having made this hypothesis he had to test it exhaustively. In twenty years he tested sixty-seven remedies on himself, family, friends and medical student volunteers. These substances were taken by many people and the results noted. The experiments were carried out under rigorous dietary and behavioural control. The noted results of major and minor symptoms were compiled into a 'Materia Medica' which, by listing what a substance could cause, was at the same time a treatise on what each substance could cure. He also wrote the first edition of 'The Organon of Medicine'. This book, the summary of his theory and philosophy, was published in 1810 and it constitutes both a remarkable exercise in logic and an enduring charter for caring medicine.

He carried on his work and investigations tirelessly but could not accumulate enough evidence of medical cures, using his system, until the winter of 1812/13 when Napoleon's army was retreating across Europe and had lost the battle of Leipzig, where Hahnemann lived. Here Hahnemann treated 180 cases of Typhus in the disease-ridden stragglers and townspeople and only two died, one of these a very old man. Later in his life, one of his students also proved the potential of this system on a large scale. In 1831 there was an epidemic of Cholera and in Raab this doctor treated 154 cases and lost six (3.9%). Orthodox doctors treating 1500 cases between them lost 821 (54.7%). These results speak for themselves. (Both episodes preceded the knowledge of bacteria or antibiotics, which raises the question whether this knowledge is vitally important for the cure of disease.)

POTENCY

The tests of substances on healthy people, 'the provings',* were only one part of his amazing discoveries. The second part was that, as he set about to find the minimum dose necessary for a cure, he found that the more dilute he made his remedies the more effective they became. This methodical serial dilution and succussion (his method of vigorously mixing the diluted remedies at each stage) he called potentisation. He wrote:

* Poorly translated from the German: Prufing – a test.

'The very smallest doses of medicines chosen for the homoeopathic diseases are each a match for the corresponding disorder. The Physician will choose a homoeopathic remedy in just so small a dose as will overcome the disease'.

Conventional medicine, whether using antiopathy (the treatment by opposites to neutralise a disease symptom) or allopathy (the treatment by an unrelated substance to try to alter the body's response to disease), is totally different in this respect. If one dilutes below the usual dose, efficacy is lost. This is clearly not so in homoeopathy. Thus Hahnemann's discovery of the ability to use infinitely dilute solutions has allowed us to use immeasurably low doses of a substance to effect a cure. We can use some of nature's most powerfully poisonous substances, such as arsenic or snake venoms, to effect most dramatic curative processes without the need to worry about potential toxicity.

ALLOPATHY AND ANTIOPATHY

Hahnemann wrote so vehemently against the illogical allopaths of his day (those that used substances unrelated to the disease) that he turned the conventional school of medical opinion drastically against him. Thus the acceptance of his theories of homoeopathy was limited. Nowadays, conventional medicine has eliminated many of those irrelevant and harmful practices from its repertoire, so it no longer needs to smart under the worst of Hahnemann's criticisms of allopathy, but it still has to contend with Hahnemann's criticisms of antiopathy. Most of modern conventional medicine (wrongly termed allopathy) is antiopathy, that is, the treatment of a disease symptom with an agent designed to neutralise or oppose that symptom. Examples of this are corticosteroids to suppress inflammation, pain killers (anodynes) to suppress pain, antitussives to suppress a cough, antiemetics to suppress vomiting, purgatives to combat constipation and binding agents to counteract diarrhoea. These medicines have a logic* but against that one has Hahnemann's arguments against

---

* Based on the principle of palliation.

suppression of symptoms and his justifications for treatment by 'like' substances. He states, and this is hard to contradict:

'Important symptoms of persistent diseases have never been treated with such palliative, antagonistic remedies without the opposite state, a relapse – indeed a palpable aggravation – of the malady occurring hours afterwards' (6th edition of the Organon).

He expands (and this observation still rings true today):–

'For a persistent tendency to sleepiness during the day the physician prescribed coffee, and when it had exhausted its action the day-somnolence increased. For frequent waking at night he gave in the evening, without heeding the other symptoms of the disease, Opium, which by virtue of its primary action produced the same night (dull, stupefied) sleep, but the subsequent nights were still more sleepless than before.'

He also uses the same logic against the antiopathic treatment of diarrhoea or constipation. This is all stated for humans but the same applies in veterinary usage. Who has not seen the suppression of a dog's itch by corticosteroid therapy and the subsequent recurrence with renewed vigour after the therapy has worn off? He even postulated that some cancers arise from continued suppression of disease symptoms. The case history (on p. 167) of the rodent ulcer illustrates a similar point.

Sadly today's conventional (antiopathic) medicine has inherited much of the discredited and obsolete allopath's suspicion and animosity towards Hahnemann's homoeopathic theory. Despite its painstakingly scientific origins, and despite Hahnemann's unerring powers of observation, modern scientific medicine cannot accept his findings. A look at contemporary medical breakthroughs shows us what a sad loss it is to us all that Hahnemann's discoveries could not have gone side by side with the scientific developments of those times, which have preceded today's conventional medicine.

The chronological list shows an increasing preoccupation with the details of scientific theory and development and, had they been coupled with Hahnemann's logic (worked out, as can be seen, way ahead of his time – his results long predating any realistic expectation of success by modern medical standards), would have given us an unparalleled composite medical theory. This is still to come if the power of scientific thought can be directed at a more realistic and appropriate analysis of hahnemannian principles.

460–375 BC (approx.)	HIPPOCRATES: Origins of a rational approach to medicine, writings rediscovered only in the Middle Ages, reputed references to theory of 'like-cures-like'.
129–200 AD	GALEN: Rational approach to anatomy – lost until 1540.
1540	VESALIUS: Builds on Galen's work.
1628	HARVEY: Theories of blood circulation.
1680's	LEEUWENHOEK: Discovery of bacteria although they were not recognised as being involved in disease.
1753	LIND: Discovery that scurvy is preventable by inclusion of fruit and fresh vegetables in diet.
1755	BIRTH OF HAHNEMANN
1755	BLACK: ⎫ Discovery of gases which make up air
1766	CAVENDISH: ⎭ (oxygen and hydrogen)
1773	HUNTER: Changes approach to surgery.
1781–1785	PRIESTLY/CAVENDISH/LAVOISIER: Discover composition of water.
1784	HAHNEMANN: First medical essay, denouncing bad medical practice of his day, praising veterinary surgeons and natural medicine.
1785–1795	FOUNDING of the veterinary profession in England.
1790	HAHNEMANN: Work on Cinchona bark, evolution of Homoeopathy.
1790	SPALLANZANI: Non-spontaneous generation of microbes (still not concerned with disease).
1790s	GROWTH OF HOMOEOPATHIC MATERIA MEDICA
1791	HUNTER: Uprating of the veterinary profession.
1793	NEW VETERINARY COLLEGE: Denounces 'quackery' in English veterinary surgery.
1795	HAHNEMANN: Essays on value of sleep, clothing, social medicine, sanitation, fresh air, fresh water, exercise and

diet; and of the ills of poverty, lack of family, education etc. (These ideas are truly holistic and were very much ahead of their time when put in this chronological list).

1796   JENNER: First vaccination (related to Isopathy?). This work has subsequently been questioned for its veracity of reporting statistics.

1810–1843   SUCCESSIVE EDITIONS OF HAHNEMANN'S 'ORGANON'.

1811–1821   SUCCESSIVE PARTS OF HAHNEMANN'S 'MATERIA MEDICA PURA' PUBLISHED.

1811   AVOGADRO: Atomic Theory.

1813   HAHNEMANN: Treatment of Typhus in Leipzig, curing an incredible 178 cases out of 180. One of those to die was a very old man. Nothing was yet known of bacterial involvement in disease nor of hygiene nor of antibiotics.

1824   DUTROCHET: See 1839.

1828   HAHNEMANN: 'Chronic diseases; their peculiar nature and their homoeopathic cure' published.

1831   OUTBREAK OF CHOLERA in Raab. Homoeopathy loses 6 out of 154 (4%). Conventional medicine of the day loses 821 out of 1501 (55%).

HAHNEMANN, with reference to the epidemic of cholera sweeping Europe, gave very advanced advice on ventilation, hygiene, infection, quarantine and sterilisation of clothing and belongings:

'In order to make the infection and spread of cholera impossible, the garments, linen etc. of all strangers have to be kept in quarantine (whilst their bodies were cleansed with speedy baths and provided with clean clothes) and retained there for two hours at stove heat of 80°C – this represents a heat at which all known infectious matters and consequently the living miasmas are annihilated.'

'The most stinking infections took place and made astounding progress whenever in the stuffy places of ships, filled as they are with musty aqueous vapours, the Cholera miasma found an element favourable to its own

multiplication and throve to an enormously increased swarm of those infinitely small, invisible living organisms which are murderously hostile to human life and which most probably form the infections matter of Cholera'.

It is surprising that Hahnemann has written a very up-to-date (although strangely worded) advisory document on the prevention of Cholera. The ideas incorporated (when put in modern language with medical jargon corrected) are well able to stand up to modern medical theory despite the fact that half a century was still to pass before the basis of that theory was laid down (Pasteur, Lister, Koch etc.). Still more surprising perhaps is that Hahnemann was able to cure by homoeopathy without recourse to those modern medical theories! He pre-empted the theories, used them for prevention and used his own homoeopathic therapeutic theory for cure. This approach should form a pattern for future human and veterinary medicine.

1833   FARADAY: Laws for electricity and magnetism.

1835   BASSI: Microbes cause disease in silkworms – his work was not widely accepted!

1837   MÜLLER: Discovers the function of nerves.

1839   SCHWANN & SCHLIEDEN: Cell theory expanded from 1824. The modern obsession with cellular chemistry may have started here.

1843   DEATH OF HAHNEMANN.

1846   MORTON: Anaesthetic ether vapour.

1853   FLORENCE NIGHTINGALE: Pioneered nursing.

1854–1856   FLORENCE NIGHTINGALE: Put theories into practice in Crimea.

1864   PASTEUR: Germ theory of disease – methods of sterilisation. Ironically Pasteur finally swayed the arguments whether germs caused disease or were incidental to disease. Homoeopathy recognises both concepts with the emphasis on the latter. Modern medicine does too but the emphasis is on the former.

1865   LISTER: Pioneered antiseptics – Carbolic.

1865   BERNARD: Principles of scientific investigation. Also theories on the body's internal environment. The start of hormone theory.

1866   MENDEL: Fundamental laws of inheritance.

1877   MANSON: Discovered the spread of disease by insect vectors.

1882   BERI BERI DISEASE: Controlled by Japanese navy by reducing rice in diet. This tied in with Lind 1753.

1882   KOCH: Discovered the Tubercle Bacillus.

1883   KOCH: Discovered the Cholera agent. (So long after Hahnemann's writings, see 1831).

1880s   PASTEUR: Vaccines for Rabies and Anthrax. This and Jenner's work were enlightened shots in the dark, viruses were yet to be discovered.

1884   KOLLER: Local anaesthetic – Cocaine.

1886   KOCH: Methods of study of bacteria, theories of vaccination and infection. These were evolved in yet another Cholera epidemic in Europe. Hahnemann's work was not used.

1887   BUIST: First sees a virus but does not recognise it for what it is (Cowpox virus).

1891   MURRAY: First hormone extract (Thyroid).

1892   IWANOWSKI: Filtrable agent caused Tobacco Mosaic disease (a step towards discovering viruses).

1895   RÖNTGEN: Discovered X-rays.

1898   BEIJERINCK: Discovered viruses.

1900   ROSS & MANSON: Proved that the Malaria parasite is spread by the mosquito. This was the disease with which Hahnemann first embarked on his homoeopathic adventure.

1902   BAYLISS & STARLING: First use of the word 'hormone'.

1900s   CURIE: Discovered Radium and its ability to suppress cancer, sterilise bacteria etc.

1903   BUCHNER: Discovered enzymes in yeast.

1906   PASCHEN: Rediscovered Small Pox virus.

1929   FLEMING: Penicillin, the first antibiotic.

1929   WOODRUFF & GOODPASTURE: Discovered Fowl Pox virus.

1931   WOODRUFF & GOODPASTURE: Culture viruses in eggs, laying down the foundation of modern virus vaccine production.

1932   KING & WAUGH: Isolated the first vitamin (C).

1935   STANLEY: Crystallised viruses.

1935   DISCOVERY OF SULPHONAMIDES in chemotherapy. This was a useful addition to Penicillin and together they still form the basis of modern antibacterial therapy.

1939   FIRST VIRUS SEEN under electron microscope.

1940   LARGE SCALE USE OF PENICILLIN commences.

Since then a horde of drugs acting at the cellular level have been discovered and manufactured. Modern medicine and homoeopathy really started to diverge in the second half of the nineteenth century owing to the deluge of scientific discoveries occurring from then onwards.

What a shame that Hahnemann and his followers, who evolved a system of medicine that required no name for a disease, no identification of bacteria or viruses and no knowledge of cellular chemistry or physiology should work in one direction while the rest of the medical world worked in a direction of the study of disease from the point of view of disease agents, cellular mechanisms and physiological and biochemical pathways.* The two were ideologically unable to work together. Much has been lost as a result and for this Hahnemann must be held jointly responsible, for he was unbridled in his attacks on conventional medical men and showed an arrogance and self-righteousness in his response to attack which could not endear him to any but devout disciples.

* See also Chapter 15 and Appendix 8.

THE WAY FORWARD

What is needed today is a selection from the best of both worlds. One needs Hahnemann's insight into the nature and mechanisms of disease, his painstaking methods and his taut principles coupled with the enquiring mind of the modern scientist. Let us look at one of Hahnemann's own comments against the illogical allopaths of his day:

> *'To render (through ignorance) if not fatal, at all events incurable, the vast majority of all diseases, namely those of a chronic charac- ter, by continually weakening and tormenting the debilitated patient, already suffering without that, from his disease and by adding new destructive drug diseases, this clearly seems to be the unhallowed main business of the old school of medicine (allopathy) and a very easy business it is when one has become an adept in this pernicious practice, and is sufficiently insensible to the stings of conscience.'*

Charming words indeed! Little wonder the medical world turned against him. Take however his positive side, betrayed by the opening paragraphs of the Organon:

> *'The physician's high and only mission is to restore the sick to health, to cure as it is termed. The highest ideal of cure is rapid, gentle and permanent restoration of health; or removal and annihil- ation of the disease in its whole extent, in the shortest, most reliable, and most harmless way on easily comprehensible principles.*
> *If the physician clearly perceives what is to be cured in diseases, if he clearly perceives what is curative in each medicine and if he knows how to adapt, according to clearly defined principles, what is curative in medicines to what he has discovered to be morbid in the patient – to adapt it as well in respect of suitability of medicines as also in respect to the proper dose and the proper period for repeat- ing the dose:– if, finally, he knows the obstacles to recovery in each case and is aware how to remove them, so that the restoration may be permanent, then he understands how to treat judiciously and rationally, and he is a true practitioner of the healing art.'*

We do well to remember those principles today whether doctors or veterinary surgeons. In fact it is encouraging to know that Hahnemann thought very highly of veterinary surgeons and their clinical prowess especially in their treatment of ulcers (still a very difficult clinical problem). He wrote:

'In spite of this my pride does not prevent me from confessing that veterinary surgeons are usually more successful, that is, have more skill in the treatment of old wounds than the most learned professors and members of the academics – I wish I had their skill based on experience, which they have frequently only acquired through treating animals.'   *(From his first essay 1784*
'Directions for curing old sores and ulcers').

The same essay – written 6 years before his discovery of homoeopathy – makes recommendation for a reversion to natural medicine:

'Their importance draws the conscientious physician more and more to simple nature amidst the rejoicing of his patients'.

It is interesting to note that ethically minded veterinary surgeons in the dawning of their official profession in England also denounced the quackery to be found in the surgery performed by the vagrant 'farrier vets' of the day. To be fair it is right to quote alongside Hahnemann's praise of veterinarians in the medicine field this vehement condemnation of some of their number in the surgery field.

'If we observe the dangerous practice of farriers, in their surgical operation, we shall see them daily sacrificing horses, by boldly mangling the original parts of the body, without knowing anything of its structure. How many muscles, and tendons, divided cross-ways, veins opened, nerves destroyed, membranes torn and essential organs more or less affected, by the ignorant boldness of these unskilled operators, whose reputation has been supported merely by public supineness and credulity!' (1791).

Strong words were obviously not Hahnemann's copyright! Happily surgery has progressed greatly since these times, thanks in great part to the work of John Hunter in the human and veterinary fields. From a homoeopath's point of view, however, because surgery has become so skilled these days, and so high-tech, it may be asked to perform too many tasks better left to effective (homoeopathic) medicine.

WHAT IS HOMOEOPATHY?

Homoeopathy is the selection of a substance, in order to cure disease in a patient, by the knowledge that the same substance is able to cause, in a healthy body, symptoms similar to those seen in the patient (see p. 1).

Also now an accepted part of Homoeopathy, is the principle of the minimal dose (see pp. 4, 203). The substances used are diluted serially, either in 1/10th stages (decimal dilutions) or 1/100th stages (centesimal dilutions), which are designated x and c potencies respectively. Thus *Arnica 30c* is a tincture of Arnica diluted one in a hundred, thirty times or a dilution of 10^{-60}. *Arnica 6x* is a tincture of Arnica diluted one in ten, six times, that is, a dilution of 10^{-6}. Succussion is carried out at each stage and it is this which seems to release the curative energy of the substance to imprint in the 'memory' of the water structure, while the successive dilution removes its toxic or harmful effects. Homoeo-pathic remedies can therefore be used in the confidence that, even if the wrong remedy is chosen, while it will achieve no cure it cannot be toxic nor cause side-effects.*

The principles governing choice of remedy are outlined in Chapter 5 and some leading guides are to be found in Chapters 8–14, so it suffices to reiterate here that, in order to gain a cure by homoeopathy, one must obtain as close a match of disease symptoms in the patient to symptoms in the materia medica as one possibly can. I will discuss the limitations this imposes on veterinary homoeopathy in Chapter 5. It is important to remember, however, that a patient exhibits a totality of symptoms whether they be behavioural, physical or mental; symptoms of the whole body or only a part of it (the so called 'generals' and 'particulars' of homoeopathy); or whether they be common symptoms or rarer 'peculiar' ones. Thus treating a patient homoeopathically implies a treatment of the whole patient not just a diseased part. This allows a patient's own individual reaction to a disease (that reaction constitutes a symptom) to influence one's choice of remedy for that

* But see footnote p 44.

patient. One does not therefore treat a named disease but the totality of symptoms representing that individual patient. Two patients with the same named disease will often be given different remedies. This individuality in response to a disease (which undoubtedly occurs) is what often confuses those thinking in the way of conventional medicine, which is reliant upon diagnosis of a named disease (a named disease is supposed to give uniform identifiable symptoms and receive uniform treatment). The picture is also confused when a conventional medicine is given, in that a patient also reacts with its own individual sensitivity to that medicine. Homoeopathy not only allows for the patient's reaction, it demands a knowledge of it.

As can be understood from the history of homoeopathy (p. 1), as a form of medicine it has depended for its data upon 'provings' in people. These people were volunteers. This has always been the case and is still going on today. Animal experimentation in the evaluation of medicines has therefore not played a part and is not necessary for the practice of human homoeopathy. This has endeared it to many who deplore the use of experimental animals in conventional medicine, whether for human or veterinary use. However, this imposes limitations on the use of homoeopathy for veterinary purposes as has been outlined in Chapter 5. This limitation is imposed by the fact that we must assume a similarity of symptoms produced by a substance, whether in humans or in different species of animals. This could hold true for most but certainly not all of our remedies, although we appear to be able to extrapolate in most cases. 'Field trials' in veterinary work, (careful trial work carried out on populations of farm animals and pets in the normal course of veterinary work, as opposed to experiments under laboratory conditions) are providing useful data while still adhering to the humane traditions of homoeopathy, but the problems of possible species differences still do apply. A knowledge of comparative toxicology aids us in this study.

MECHANISM OF HOMOEOPATHY

Since one is using a remedy similar in its action to the disease itself and since the principle isolated in the remedy is probably a form of energy,

owing to the dilution/succussion process (potentisation), the homoeopathic remedy most probably acts upon the body's system in the same
way as the disease but in a more powerful manner eclipsing the disease.
If one takes the homoeopath's view that disease (literally dis-ease or
ill-at-ease) is a dynamic disturbance of the body (rather than an entity
in itself as conventional medicine implies) then what could be better as
a cure than a remedy of purely dynamic quality? Since it is thought
that a homoeopathic medicine is only energetic in nature, its effect in
the body is unlikely to last forever and is therefore easily dissipated
from the system, so that its own disease-producing ability is never
realised. (See Chapter 6 figs 2–6 for further thoughts on this subject.)
I quote from Samuel Hahnemann:

> '*A weaker dynamic affection is permanently extinguished in the
> living organism by a stronger one, if the latter (whilst differing in
> kind) is very similar to the former in its manifestations.*'

He goes on eloquently and logically (as always) to establish why
homoeopathic medicines are more powerful than the disease agents
they are employed to combat.

The homoeopath's theory of disease and its cure is therefore lifted
straight from the writings of Samuel Hahnemann. He postulated:

a) A vital force within a patient.
b) A disease as a morbid influence upon that vital force.
c) The symptoms as an expression of the reaction of that vital force
   to disease influence.
d) An effective medicine as one which mimics those symptoms when
   applied to the vital force.
e) The medicine as a more powerful influence than the disease,
f) which stimulates the vital force to overpower the disease, thus
   unleashing the vital force's full power to extinguish the new
   temporary influence and restore the patient to health.

An analogy can be drawn with a comparison between brute force
and judo as methods of self-defence.

To apply a force opposite to the aggressor, if the aggressor is strong,
will fail, whereas if only one applies a force in the same direction as the

aggressor (the art of judo) a very powerful adversary can be defeated with small and economical use of force. This, superficially, is the strength of homoeopathy.

The homoeopath's concept of cure of disease may be summarised:

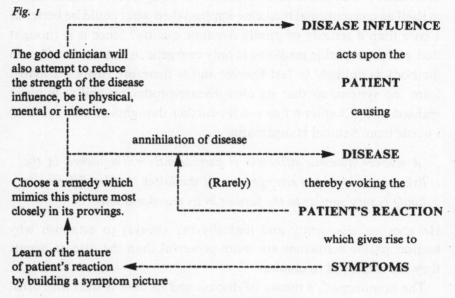

Fig. 1

DISEASE INFLUENCE

The good clinician will also attempt to reduce the strength of the disease influence, be it physical, mental or infective.

acts upon the

PATIENT

causing

annihilation of disease

DISEASE

Choose a remedy which mimics this picture most closely in its provings.

(Rarely)

thereby evoking the

PATIENT'S REACTION

which gives rise to

Learn of the nature of patient's reaction by building a symptom picture

SYMPTOMS

Dotted lines are disease-mitigating pathways. (See also p. 115.)

RATIONAL DISCUSSION OF COMMON CRITICISMS OF THE HOMOEOPATHIC METHOD

1 It is argued that homoeopaths do not understand how their remedies work so how can they, as scientifically trained professional people, use them? It can be said that, once having accepted that what a substance can cause it can also cure then one can postulate the way a homoeopathic remedy works. It is thought to work by mimicking exactly, or very closely, the dynamic disease process in the body and thereby stimulating such a powerful reaction in the body similar to that evoked by the disease influence that the body overpowers the disease. The remedy, being only energy, then fades and the body is cured of its disease process; the symptoms then cease. This does not constitute knowledge or full understanding but how much more can it

be said that we fail to understand the workings of modern drugs? Who can foretell the side effects of new drugs? Who can predict what new disease can be introduced by the use of biological medicines, stray material from vaccines and organ or tissue transplants (or even transgenic implants)? Who can divine the potential for harm in genetic engineering and other forms of biotechnology? Drugs and chemicals are often tested in unrelated species. Homoeopathic remedies for the human are tested in humans. They can be tested, on a humane basis, in animals too, for the benefit of animals.

2   It is argued that so-called cures by homoeopathic treatments are not proven, because:

a) They are not evaluated in proper trials,
b) The condition could have self-cured at the same time as the homoeopathic treatment was applied,
c) The diagnosis could have been incorrect.

We may respond rationally by saying:

a) Clinical trials are in progress in man and animals, under field conditions, and are proving very promising. Many existing results are very convincing.
b) There are too many coincidences of this kind to accept this hypothesis for the curing of so many cases. This and the next argument could just as easily be levelled at any form of medicine, including the conventional system. Furthermore, many cases have proved to be of a chronic nature prior to homoeopathic involvement and have long persisted despite previous conventional efforts. Why should they suddenly and spontaneously resolve coincidental with the timing of homoeopathic input? That would defy reason and logic.
c) The diagnosis can always be incorrect since human judgement is involved. However, taking a great many cases where orthodox clinicians have satisfied themselves with a diagnosis indicating surgery, incurability or euthanasia, apparent cures have been effected by use of homoeopathy. The diagnosis could still have been wrong since no clinician is infallible but the orthodox

clinician was satisfied to the extent that euthanasia or surgery would have been carried out but for homoeopathic intervention.

3   It is often said that the doses used ensure that no material substance is present in the remedy, therefore no cure is possible. Here one can only ask: What do we know of what is curative in a substance? Need it be a material part of that substance or could it be, for instance, an energy pattern derived from that substance? Again trial work shows that there is an effect so we need to rethink our ideas on drug mechanisms to suit the new evidence. Since science cannot yet explain the phenomenon, science has some learning still to do.

4   The placebo effect is often said to be the mechanism behind the apparent cures. This is the means whereby a patient can be cured by the psychological benefit of receiving a treatment, whatever that treatment may be. In other words the patient is humoured to such an extent by receiving a treatment, however ineffective or inapplicable, that his body's mechanisms effect a self-cure. This could be true in humans in some cases but surely is unlikely to occur in animals (and certainly not in animals dosed via their drinking water, who don't even know they are being treated!) and therefore the practice of veterinary homoeopathy has countered this criticism. It is an interesting point that those who condemn homoeopathy as having no demonstrable mechanism can accept the strange and wonderful phenomenon of the placebo effect without question. Surely the placebo effect (a well-proven phenomenon) is proof enough of the body's mysterious healing powers? Secondly homoeopathic treatment often works in cases when other treatments have failed. Surely, were the placebo effect the mechanism here, then it should have operated already, prior to the homoeopathic treatment?

5   It is said that homoeopathy is not levelled at the supposed root cause of the disease e.g. bacteria, or the cellular or humoral mechanisms involved in the disease process, and therefore has no hope of achieving a cure. Here again, if one hypothesises that disease is not necessarily caused by bacteria, etc., but that these in many cases may be incidental to disease and opportune invaders and that deviations of

cellular and humoral pathways are but a part of the symptoms of (that is, the patient's reaction to) the disease then why does one need to focus one's attentions upon them so closely, however interesting such a study might be? Treat the patient and nourish, guide and stimulate the 'vital force' and these symptoms and opportune invaders will perish. The real cause of disease goes much deeper, it is the fundamental imbalance of the organism (and the forces that create that imbalance) and homoeopathy does address and treat that real cause.

6 It can be said, perhaps that a patient coming to a homoeopathic physician has faith in that physician and therefore a cure results. The same argument applies as in number 4. Animals surely disprove this theory.

7 It could be argued that homoeopathic remedies, unbeknown to the homoeopath, contain an impurity which is an accidental curative agent applicable to the disease in question.

a) Homoeopathic pharmacies are under just as strict governmental legislative control as are conventional pharmacies. Quality control and batch tracing are normal practice, so such effects become unlikely.

b) As can be seen in Chapters 8–14, the remedies are successfully used, each against a wide spectrum of symptoms. Surely no accidental ingredient could achieve the results claimed of the correctly chosen homoeopathic remedy against such a wide variety of seemingly unrelated symptoms in 'unrelated' organs? Secondly the same accidental ingredient would be very unlikely to appear in all batches of any one remedy therefore one would be totally unable to achieve consistent results, were an accidental ingredient the effective portion. Thirdly, why would a remedy chosen by the similia principle appear to work, when an irrelevant remedy fails, if it is only an accidental ingredient which is effective? This ingredient should by law of averages appear in any remedy and therefore any remedy is just as likely to work.

None of these rational arguments is intended to decry conventional antiopathic medicine. They are all intended to infuse the essential ingredient of logic into any discussion on homoeopathy. By careful logic alone should we be guided in our research for the ultimate healing truth. This must be our quest if we are to aspire to Hahnemann's idea of a physician's mission (p. 11).

WHY USE HOMOEOPATHY?

This chapter has not served its purpose at all if it has not shown the peculiarities of homoeopathy that make it a very sensible choice of treatment in animals whenever the similia principle can be established. The following points can serve to reiterate its main points:–

1 No side effects (see p. 44 and p. 53 however).

2 No suppression of symptoms and signs, for later more vicious reappearance.

3 No dependence upon diagnosis in the purely conventional sense but more a dependence upon accurate and exhaustive observation of signs and symptoms, including if necessary X-ray, blood sample and other 'symptoms'.

This not only allows one to treat animals suffering an undiagnosable disease, but also enables one to tackle any new disease, as yet not classified in terms of agents and suggested treatments. Recent cases in point are Parvo-virus in dogs and Key-Gaskell Syndrome in cats,* which homoeopathy was able to help prior to the official recognition of the diseases.

4 No need for laboratory experiments on animals for the testing of medicines.

5 Allowance for and dependence upon a patient's individuality.

6 Whole patient treatment; it is often said in the consulting room, after a course of homoeopathic treatment, that the patient has *never been better*. This implies a deeper effect of the remedy than one

* At time of 1st Edition.

might expect, acting upon the whole patient not just upon the superficial symptoms of disease. (The holistic concept is justified by this phenomenon.)

7 Homoeopathy appears to work with and encourage the body's own disease-combating mechanisms to effect a cure and this constitutes a most natural, humane and effective method of cure.

8 No environmental pollution.

9 Ability to treat the foetus in utero preventing the effects of illness of the dam and miasmatic effects. (A possible interpretation of the word Eugenics.)

10 In farm animals, no residues of medicines in milk, meat, eggs etc.

Now please read on and enjoy the following chapters which attempt to act as a guide to the practical use of homoeopathic remedies in the veterinary application. Please may I exhort you all to purchase *Arnica* and use it according to the guidelines described in the relevant parts of Chapters 8–14, in order firstly to obtain a feel for the use of homoeopathic remedies. (*Arnica* is so frequently indicated that one will be using it often), and secondly to convince yourself of the far-reaching and often astonishing effects of homoeopathy upon the expected course of the conditions described, had you not used the remedy. I also refer you to page 32, Chapter 3, in this connection.

CHAPTER 2

When to Call the Vet

Not for nothing have veterinarians undergone five or six years of rigorous training. Their accumulated knowledge on the variability, scope and effect of disease, their ability to assess seriousness of a case, their ability to institute such correct dietary, supportive, nursing and management procedures as can aid a cure are all to be greatly respected, *whether or not they practise homoeopathy*. It is also notably difficult to be objective about one's own family and the same applies to one's own pets. The veterinarian can provide the valuable objectivity needed. I commend you to re-read Hahnemann's words quoted on p. 11 taken from the opening paragraphs of the Organon. These words call for a high level of dedication and understanding. Only by persistent practice, constant reading, repeated harsh lessons of experience and by encountering the sheer variety of reaction to disease shown by a multiplicity of patients are veterinarians able to be aware of what is to be cured in disease (that is noticing all the symptoms). Only by these same lessons and experiences can they be aware of what is curative in medicines (that is, the 'provings' in the Materia Medica). Only by constant practice can they learn to match symptoms to provings, choose the correct remedy, dose at the required level, at the required frequency for an adequate duration. Only through training and experience can he or she learn the nursing and management tricks necessary to 'removing the obstacles to recovery'. Although Hahnemann is talking about the practice of homoeopathy, conventional veterinary medicine should also have much to offer in this respect and owners should not lightly undertake the treatment of their own animals unless they feel competent to assess the seriousness of the case unaided.

This is not to say that pet owners, safe in the knowledge that homoeopathic medicines have no side effects, cannot usefully set to work to treat their own pets, using guidelines set down in this book and using the handy reference chapters on disease syndromes and remedies (Chapters 8–14). However, what they must try to do is to be aware of what is dangerous in the way of disease and what is not dangerous, what is serious and what is not so serious, what is acute and what is chronic, what may benefit from veterinary help and what absolutely requires it, what requires immediate action and what is not so desperate. All this seems to be asking rather a lot but most of it should be instinctive. One must learn how to let instincts come to the surface of awareness. Those who have experience of children and their ailments should know what is meant by all these considerations. An infant is very similar in the problems set for parent and doctor to a pet and the problems it sets for carer and veterinarian. The dramatic effect upon the demeanour of child or pet by acute disease, the lack of verbal communication about symptoms, the concern felt by parent or pet-carer, all are very similar. Since so many people have contact with infants in health and sickness this should given them confidence to deal more certainly with their pet's ailments. The human race has deeply rooted instincts in relation to management of disease in its children. These should be given full rein when it comes to considering one's pets' problems.

In Chapters 8–14, those conditions where veterinary help should most certainly be sought are marked as such. Other conditions can reasonably be considered for treatment at home. Also remember that no condition is so serious that a home remedy, immediately administered prior to veterinary attention, cannot be of benefit and support. Although, in many cases, subsequent conventional veterinary medicine can counteract a homoeopathic remedy given at home, there are no cases where a homoeopathic remedy can conflict with the subsequent conventional treatment to the detriment of the patient. This knowledge should encourage immediate home first aid medicine.

Now to apply logic to determine the kind of conditions wherein homoeopathy alone should not be used, whether by veterinarian or pet carer. This is not to say that homoeopathy cannot help in such cases, it almost certainly can, since most of these conditions do not confine their effect to the locality of the body in which they occur but have a general effect as well. Consider them in more detail and this will become clear.

The first type to be considered are those rare conditions in which a bacterial infection is running its course in such a violent manner as to render the 'vital force' more or less unable to fight back. If a homoeopathic remedy alone is used under these circumstances – however correct that remedy might be – the condition may proceed unabated, owing to the tremendous hold the bacterial infection has e.g. meningitis, acute septicaemia, leptospiral jaundice. If however the appropriate antibiotic is given (the domain of the veterinarian who alone understands the factors affecting choice and administration of these medicines) the downward trend in the patient can be temporarily reversed, releasing the 'vital force' from this stranglehold and leaving room for the appropriate homoeopathic remedy to effect a complete and lasting cure. In this manner one is using (as suggested in the introduction to this book) the best of both worlds. One cannot, in one's right mind, adhere to homoeopathy and shut out modern scientific developments to the detriment of the patient and not be accused of gross folly or neglect. It is possible that those who are totally proficient in homoeopathy can minimise the use of antibiotic or do without it altogether but *unless one has that skill and confidence* the patient must not be jeopardised.

Another set of circumstances where one may not be able to sit back and leave it to homoeopathy alone is the realm of injury. Again there are valuable homoeopathic remedies which can be relied upon to restore health in cases of minor injury (see Chapters 8–14) and help tremendously in cases of major injury (who can deny the marvellous effects of *Arnica* for instance?) but again one would be sadly neglecting one's duty if one failed to staunch the flow of blood from a wound by appropriate methods, stitch a large wound to aid healing, immobilize a fracture or severe strain to prevent pain and further damage, remove an injurious foreign body (if this action is necessary to recovery), replace dislocations, use surgery to repair any internal damage that is preventing recovery or institute measures to prevent any external influence which can impede the healing process. If one fails to do these one fails to fulfil the resolutions laid down on p. 11 of Chapter 1. It would do no harm to read these resolutions again now. A veterinarian is bound by these as rules of the profession but a pet carer who takes upon himself the medicinal care of a pet must also take these resolutions to heart, calling for help when needed. He becomes, for the moment, the 'physician' to whom Hahnemann refers, but must know when to refer the patient to a qualified veterinarian for more specialised help.

A third circumstance where, again, one should not lean entirely on homoeopathy, is the field of necessary surgery. Congenital reparable defects should be repaired by the appropriate surgical method if they constitute a threat to the animal's health. Abdominal catastrophes must be dealt with in the appropriate manner e.g. a swallowed foreign body (many cannot pass), intussusception (many will not self correct), abdominal adhesions which produce malfunction of the bowel and many other circumstances of a like nature. (Physiological dysfunction of the bowel can probably be corrected non-surgically by the appropriate homoeopathic methods.) Cancerous growths should only be removed if they constitute an immediate threat to health or life (rather than rely on homoeopathy to cure such growths) at the same time using a homoeopathic remedy to correct the state of the 'vital force' which is predisposed to this condition in the first place. Removal of a cancerous growth is dangerous because it removes the ability of the clinician to monitor the disease and may excite secondary growths. It is therefore a technique to be reserved only as an emergency life-saver or to 'buy time'. There may be no substitute to surgery to correct anatomical defects bred into an animal by successive malpractice of some early animal breeders. Such hereditary defects include ear or eye deformities of spaniels and blood hounds and leg deformities of many miniature breeds. It goes without saying, if a veterinarian meets such conditions in a breeding establishment, that he will do all in his power to influence that breeder and others to try to eliminate the condition by good breeding practice and will only correct such conditions surgically if it is to the benefit of the animal in question to do so.

It is sometimes necessary, as a last resort, to institute major surgery such as castration or ovarohysterectomy to correct a condition which fails (for whatever reason) to respond to homoeopathy but again the appropriate homoeopathic remedy will prove an invaluable aid to recovery. Such surgical procedures may be forced upon us by the very act of domestication which brings an animal out of its natural environment and evolved social structure, so leading to intractable physical, physiological or psychological, sexually-oriented problems.

It is not always necessary to resort to surgery to correct dental problems or urethral obstruction or to relieve severe impacted constipation by mechanical means, a homoeopathic remedy may effect a cure; but undue delay or home experimentation is not to be encouraged. These conditions can be very serious if left unrelieved, especially in the case of urinary obstruction.

In nearly all cases of surgery, another non-homoeopathic procedure is required, that of anaesthesia. In this procedure one unashamedly resorts to chemical usage, with all its attendant risks and side effects, for humane reasons. It is in fact illegal to carry out surgery without appropriate anaesthesia and rightly so in the light of medical knowledge. Acupuncture can act as a substitute for anaesthetic agents and is often used in China but is little used in this country or the rest of the world as yet. Homoeopathy can be used to lessen the side effects and after effects of anaesthetics, and should be used for this purpose. One day acupuncture may supersede some use of chemical anaesthesia in animals but there are difficulties not met in the human sphere.

Fluid therapy is often used as a support to a failing system, where rehydration or rebalancing is required. While the use of a correct homoeopathic remedy may well do away with the need for this technique in many cases, it should not be relied upon in every case and there are occasions in which the urgency of the situation prevents the home prescriber from finding the correct homoeopathic remedy in time.

When the vital force seems to be no longer able to fight a disease influence in aged animals, and a terminal situation has been reached, then exploitation of the undoubted palliative effects of drugs may be justified if there is still a chance for reasonable quality of life thereby. The risk of side effects of drugs in these sad situations is a more academic consideration, since life is not expected to be long (and the dangers of side-effects have to be less than those of euthanasia!).

The author hopes in this chapter to have illustrated the place of veterinary advice, the place of veterinary skills and the place of non-homoeopathic methods. One is left, in the final instance, to make one's own decision whether or not to consult a veterinarian but one must remember *when in doubt – consult*. Veterinarians often ask the advice of colleagues too! The most important single contribution the veterinarian is able to make for you and your pet is his or her ability to carry out a full examination, including objective observation and evaluation of symptoms and history. The veterinary training and experience give a tremendous lead over anyone who tries to do this without the advantage of such training. This capacity must not be underestimated. If it is humanly possible to avoid the mistreatment and mismanagement of a case resulting from failure to notice important symptoms, then it is more likely that a veterinarian will avoid these errors than the untrained, however enlightened and intelligent, lay person. To illustrate these points further I refer you to Chapters 4/5/6.

It is not my place to discuss veterinary professional ethics in this book but it is worth reminding both homoeopathic veterinary surgeons and pet owners that homoeopathic medicine in animals is still veterinary medicine even if it uses no drugs as we understand the word. A case referred to a homoeopathic veterinary surgeon after conventional treatment still requires, for the good of the patient, the customary inter-veterinary communication. Otherwise one fails in one's duty to learn all one can of the patient and its history. It is also to be recommended that veterinary surgeons do not yield to the temptation, put in their paths by distance, to prescribe *without first seeing the patient* so that one can, in the best veterinary and homoeopathic traditions, extract as much information from the history-taking sessions as possible. There are, sadly, still times when homoeopathy fails to achieve a cure. This is almost certainly due not so much to the patient's failure to respond to homoeopathy but more to one's inability to read correctly all the symptoms and history. I refer you to Chapter 5 on selection of remedy to explain this statement and the limitations imposed on veterinary homoeopathy by the animal's inability to talk! This makes it very important to use one's diagnostic ability to the utmost and distance is not conducive to increasing one's chances of success.

If you wish to visit a veterinarian using homoeopathy it is advisable to ascertain whether that veterinarian is well enough versed in homoeopathy to be able to take on the particular problem and species concerned. When visiting a veterinarian for a homoeopathic second opinion it will be necessary to provide a full case history from your own original veterinarian. The homoeopathic colleague will then write back to the referring veterinarian. This is a routine course of action for veterinarians and they are obliged to help you in this way.

CHAPTER 3

Getting Started

So far this book has served to show some of the scope of homoeopathy in animal disease and to encourage its use by both veterinarian and pet carer. It is possible, also, that it has left a fear of the unknown, a reluctance to 'get the feet wet' both for vet and owner. This natural hesitation is important for it shows that one has the necessary humility for the difficult task of medicine. Do not succumb to hesitancy however, but resolve to set out on the path of discovery. Purchase a few remedies (see Appendix 9), or just *Arnica* if one alone is all one dares and, using the following pages, get down to business. If, however, more help is needed there are many official bodies, publications, retailers, libraries and advisors to whom one can turn. Some useful addresses are listed at the back of this book.

The Faculty of Homoeopathy aims to advance the principles and practice of homoeopathy and works in close conjunction with the Homoeopathic Trust for Research and Education. These bodies are a source of untiring inspiration, encouragement and help to all professional people. They are central to British homoeopathy and veterinarians should always be ready to consult one or other body. There are regular courses in veterinary homoeopathy, accredited by the Faculty of Homoeopathy and these are an invaluable aid to the veterinary homoeopath as much as to the aspiring physician, along-side whom veterinarians are taught. Tutors are usually provided for further extra-curricular guidance if necessary. The British Association of Homoeopathic Veterinary Surgeons more specifically sets out to help veterinarians in their education and practice. This Association will also help in the location of veterinarians who use homoeopathy, upon receipt of SAE. The British Homoeopathic Association is a charity which exists to promote homoeopathy for both humans and animals and is a mine of useful information.

At the local level there are groups of interested lay people deeply involved in helping one to understand this complex form of medicine. They organise speakers and meetings on all aspects of the subject of homoeopathy. They are a rallying point for those wishing to further the cause of homoeopathy and an invaluable local communication medium. Much is to be learnt by attending these groups. Their titles and addresses can be obtained from the National Association of Homoeopathic Groups.

Books on the subject of homoeopathy can be bought or ordered through book shops but the Faculty of Homoeopathy, the British Homoeopathic Association and local groups all retail most of the books published. A short bibliography and further reading section is to be found in the Appendix to this book. It is worthwhile stressing again at this point the need for deep and wide reading in order to gain any degree of competence in the practice of veterinary homoeopathy. Much of the available literature may not seem relevant to veterinarians wishing to deepen their experience, or to pet carers following their interest in the subject, but be assured that, without the variety of reading to be found amongst the titles mentioned and other books omitted for the sake of conciseness, one's ability to achieve good results in the practice of homoeopathy is sadly limited. Each author has tried to pass on his or her own experiences and each reference therefore serves as a means of widening one's own experience. Reference to the treatments in Chapter 8–14 of this book alone or to any other veterinary book alone will only serve to narrow one's sphere of activity and eventually lead to the disillusionment of those who expect to do great things with homoeopathy.

Two aspects are of utmost importance when reading. The first is the gathering of homoeopathic principles. Much is written on the human medical side in this field, but sadly the principles of veterinary homoeopathy have been relatively neglected. It is for this reason that this book has devoted a great part of its content to the study of principles alone. Chapters 1–7 are dedicated to the study of the essence and principles of homoeopathy in general and veterinary homoeopathy in particular, without which study one is left as a ship without navigation; how should one proceed and by what route, to arrive at one's required destination?

The second aspect to be considered, when widening one's reading, is the practice of homoeopathy. Again a book such as this is able to supply a great deal of useful information to guide one in the practice of homoeopathic treatment of a wealth of conditions in pets which one can readily recognise. It cannot, however, cover all eventualities. It cannot approach the subject from every direction nor give a great number of different slants to the ways of recognising symptoms in animals. It cannot cover every homoeopathic medicine. For these reasons one again arrives at the conclusion that the wider the reading the greater one's flexibility and ability to detect, identify and treat successfully those deviations from the normal which we call illness.

Do not restrict your reading to animal material alone. Human material is vastly more varied and prolific and is valid to your study within the limitations laid down in Chapter 5. One should try to approach the homoeopathic treatment of animals more from a study of totality of symptoms than from a knowledge of diseases and their names and in this I hope the reader will be helped by the pages of this book and by a study of much of the human literature in the Appendix.

Nothing more now remains but to embark upon homoeopathic treatment of animals. I refer you again to Chapter 1, last paragraph, before you start and I would also like to add, at this point, some advice given to my mother before she started using veterinary homoeopathy, and which she subsequently handed on to me when I started:– 'Refer repeatedly to the books on homoeopathic materia medica (and any book which has a section on this subject) and hold in your mind as good a "picture" as you can of a few important remedies. One day a patient will come into the surgery with a classic manifestation of one of these pictures and you can then use the remedy with an unerring certainty of its applicability (by symptom match) in that case.' The rapid and effective working of the remedy under these ideal conditions is a sure way of boosting your confidence in the ability of homoeo-pathic remedies to act as they are claimed to act.

For those veterinarians who are keen to undertake a fuller study of veterinary homoeopathy and to obtain recognition for this, the Faculty of Homoeopathy administers an examination, requiring minimum attendance at accredited courses before sitting. Passing the examination entitles the candidate to use the qualification Veterinary Member of the Faculty of Homoeopathy (VetMFHom) which is the first qualification in veterinary homoeopathy in the world. The British Association of Homoeopathic Veterinary Surgeons and the Faculty of Homoeopathy can both provide a list of such qualified veterinary homoeopaths. There is also, in the pipeline at the time of writing, a more basic certificate likely to be available to veterinarians. The Faculty has yet to finalise details but it is likely to certify a preliminary understanding of veterinary homoeopathy, better enabling veterin-arians to apply first aid homoeopathy and better to understand when to refer to someone more experienced in more complex cases.

From where should one now obtain these homoeopathic medicines? It is not the place of this book to advertise manufacturers from whom one can obtain homoeopathic remedies, but addresses are available from the sources of advice to which I have referred in this chapter. A small range of low-potency medicines is also available from health shops and pharmacies around the country.

Please now resist the temptation to jump to Chapter 8 but read the intervening chapters first, in order to gain a fuller understanding of how to put your acquired principles into practice. Without a sound grounding in homoeopathic philosophy and methodology, success in therapy will be more elusive to the prescriber.

CHAPTER 4

Putting Principles into Practice 1
Taking the History in the Veterinary Clinic

Before consulting Chapters 8–14 a word of warning must be issued. This has been said in earlier chapters in a different way but must now be reiterated. Selecting a homoeopathic remedy does not consist entirely of consulting Chapter 8 and perhaps checking in Chapter 17 and leaving it at that. The remedies conveniently placed against those conditions described in Chapters 8–14 are only some of the many remedies which have been found to be of merit in treating such conditions. Some are so likely to be effective in most cases that a note is made to that effect but the majority of the remedies are not the sole recommended treatment. They are simply remedies commonly used in those contexts. If the notes match fairly closely the symptoms presented by the patient the likelihood is that they will work but if the match is not so accurate it is not advisable to 'try it anyway' but more useful to go back to square one.* In this and the next two chapters the logical sequence from square one shall be followed: Taking the history, selecting the remedy, managing the case.

TAKING THE HISTORY

Taking the history of a case is extremely important in homoeopathic veterinary medicine requiring little adaptation on the conventional veterinary surgeon's part. It does however require a modification of attitude and scope and a much greater time allowance. It is the

---

* See also Chapter 5 and Appendix 8.

essential basis for choosing a homoeopathic remedy since, in taking an accurate, and hopefully full, history one can present a logical list of symptoms to which to match the remedy. The order may be important since it matches the layout of some of the repertories and materia medica (see book list). It is worthwhile trying to establish a firm routine when taking your history and it is this which occupies the extra time which a homoeopathic consultation takes as compared with a conventional one. However, do not allow this routine to be so inflexible as to interrupt an owner's train of thought or line of conversation. You can always catch up on points later if you make a note in the margin to do so.

Introduction to Patient

1 a) Observe behaviour in the waiting room
   b) Observe entry to consulting room
   These can tell you so much about the animal and are opportunities not to be wasted. Note all the points down and refer to No. 12 later. In the case of cats the removal from the basket can be a telling time. It is even possible in some veterinary clinics to observe a dog coming out of the vehicle in which it arrived. This can also be very telling about a dog's will and its relationship with its human companion.

The Complaint

2 *What is the presenting complaint?*
   This will be the reason your client has brought the patient in to see you. *Note your client's words.*
3 *Characteristics of each symptom or sign.*
   Difficult in an animal but still very important. What sort of diarrhoea (character, colour etc.?) What sort of discharge? What type of lesion? etc.
4 *The so-called modalities.*
   What makes each symptom or sign worse? What makes it better? e.g. weather, temperature, food, drink, rest, motion.

5 *Periodicity.*

When is each symptom or sign worse or when is it better? e.g. seasons, time of day.

6 *Duration of complaint.*

How long has it been going on? When exactly did it start?

7 *Circumstances at start.*

The client may well say the patient has never been right since (for example) disease, injury, new puppy came into family, family member died, vaccination, etc.

8 *Concomitant symptoms or signs.*

If sneeze is there a nasal discharge? What sort? If diarrhoea, does the animal strain or not? Are there other seemingly unrelated symptoms or signs?

The Patient

9 *Past medical history.*

Previous treatments, vaccinations, other complaints, etc. (This is one of the many good reasons for communicating with the previous veterinary surgeon in cases of second opinion.)

10 *Family history if known.*

Easier in dog or cat breeding homes than in the average pet's home, although some information may be known.

11 *Home environment.*

e.g. working dog? Stresses caused by children in family or other pets? Broken home? 'Child' companion gone to university?

12 *Mental symptoms or signs.*

a) 'Understanding' type.

Reaction to criticism, consolation, fuss, noise, surrounding activity?

b) 'Will/Manner' type.

Dominant/submissive, aggressive/shy, neat/scruffy, careful/clumsy, impulsive/steady, memory, emotion.

13 *General symptoms or signs.*

Desires/aversions, physique, posture, gait, sleep, dreams, appetite, thirst, diet, drugs, meals (before/after?), oestrus period (before/

after?), effect on the patient of geography, season, time, temperature, weather.

14 *Particular symptoms or signs.*

This is the full examination of the animal. Note, along with symptoms or signs found in each organ system examined, the modalities as per No. 4: <>* with temperature, season, time, weather, moisture, position. etc.

The examination should encompass the entire body in a routine order preferably matched to the text in the materia medica and repertories which you use most often, e.g.: Head, Face, Eyes, Ears, Nose, Mouth, Digestive, Urinary, Female/Male, Respiratory, Heart, Circulatory and Blood, Locomotor, Lymphatic System, Nervous System and Skin.

15 *Strange and peculiar symptoms/signs.*

Special note should be taken of any strange or peculiar habit, behaviour or sign of disease, since such signs are especially applicable to *this* patient at *this* time. Hahnemann rightly asks us to place great emphasis on such phenomena in paragraph 153 of the Organon (see p. 38).

During the examination one must be highly observant, constantly using one's eyes, ears, nose and touch to ascertain all the details. It is extremely important to give weight to everything said during the consultation. Encourage discussion on anything about the patient however insignificant or foolish it may seem, being careful not to put words into an owner's mouth nor to ask leading questions or those questions just requiring an unrevealing answer 'yes' or 'no'.

From the history-taking, *'obstacles to recovery'* should come to light. They could be nutritional or dietary (q.v.), environmental, historical (q.v.) or medical. Emotions, drugs, deficiencies, dehydration, unimmobilised fractures, old disease, foreign bodies, vaccination (q.v.), etc. may each represent obstacles in any particular case.

---

* < denotes 'worse for', > denotes 'better for'.

CHAPTER 5

Putting Principles into Practice 2
Selecting the Remedy

This chapter deals alone with the actual mechanics of selection. That this chapter is so small a part of the whole, reflects the importance of the principles behind selection, relative to the actual mechanics of selection. For those of you who have jumped straight to this chapter please read no further before you read the earlier part of the book. This sounds to be very imperious advice but is worthwhile since many pitfalls of prescription can be avoided by taking into account the principles discussed in the earlier chapters and introduction. The selection of the remedy ideally suited to the case depends primarily upon the taking of an accurate and full history, therefore it will be necessary constantly to refer to Chapter 4 throughout this chapter.

I have repeatedly stated that homoeopathy is the selection of a remedy to match the patient's reaction to disease (i.e. the symptoms). What material does one need in order to do this?

Referring you again to Hahnemann's words on p. 11, clearly what is needed is:

a) The history or nature of the case. The list of symptoms under logical headings.
b) The nature of the medicines again listed under logical headings similar to those in the history (see also p. 115).

The first requirement we have just seen how to obtain by following the advice in Chapter 4. The second body of information is contained in Chapter 17 and in the various books on materia medica listed in the Appendix. A guide to where to look in materia medica is given in repertories (books listing symptoms of each part of the body with commonly applicable remedies alongside).

A short cut to this process is to use 'ready reckoners' – lists of diseases and suggested remedies worked out by experienced practitioners of the art. These can be found in the human literature and several books on the veterinary side. This book compromises in this respect, containing such a list combined with brief general considerations of symptoms such as are found in a repertory (Chapter 8). Using such lists will obviously be very much easier than using Hahnemann's first principles, but it cannot lead to such a good success rate because no writer can give, in such a list, all conditions affecting your choice of remedy under all circumstances of disease. Beware of taking too many short cuts and use ready reckoners only as a guide and *aide memoire* (see Appendix 8 and p. 41).

HAHNEMANNIAN METHOD

Hahnemann's 'Materia Medica Pura' published between 1811 and 1821 contained the provings of 66 remedies. I quote from the 6th edition of the Organon paragraph 153 which clearly shows his emphasis upon the individuality of both patient and remedy and upon detail of symptoms:

'In this search for a homoeopathic specific remedy, that is to say, in the comparison of the collective symptoms of the natural disease with the list of symptoms of known medicines, in order to find among these an artificial morbific agent corresponding by similarity to the disease to be cured, the more striking, singular, uncommon and peculiar (characteristic) signs and symptoms of the case of the disease are chiefly and most solely to be kept in view; for it is more particularly these that very similar ones in the list of symptoms of the selected remedy must correspond to, in order to constitute it the most suitable for effecting the cure. The more general and undefined symptoms:– loss of appetite, headache, debility, restless sleep, discomfort and so forth demand but little attention when of that vague and indefinite character, if they cannot be more accurately

described, as symptoms of such a general nature are observed in almost every disease and from almost every drug.'

He also set great store by the mental symptoms displayed in any illness as these most clearly represent the patient's individual response to disease. How difficult it would be with no other guide than the materia medica to match one of 66 remedies to the observed disease. How much more difficult it is now with several thousand from which to choose. Clearly the more one knows by constant reading the easier it is to match remedy to disease but thankfully there are numerous repertories to help.

REPERTORISING

The basic use of repertories I will illustrate by reference to 'Kent's Repertory with Word Index'. Under the headings of the different parts of the body Kent has listed symptoms with their modalities. Against these he has put names of remedies found to possess these same properties. Those remedies most commonly or strongly possessing these symptoms are in heavy black type, those less so in italics and those least frequently or least strongly in ordinary type. To take a symptom such as corneal opacity from an injury one can look under: 'EYE, SYMPTOMS FROM INJURY' (Kent p. 244):

Black letters: **Symphytum.**
Italics: *Arnica, Euphrasia, Ledum, Staphysagria*
Ordinary type: Aconite, Calcarea carb., Calcarea sulph, Hamamelis, Silica, Sulphur, Sulph. acid.

From this information one would be very confident prescribing *Symphytum* if no further homework were done. However, if one looks in Kent under 'EYE, OPACITY FROM WOUNDS' (Kent p. 247) one finds *Euphrasia* in italics. If, therefore, one looks into each detailed symptom one obtains a more accurate matching. The more symptoms identified and cross-referenced, the more accurate the match. At the end of this process, a short list of possible remedies must be carefully checked in a Materia Medica for the closest match to the patient *in totality*. This method has even lent itself to computerisation in the present day, which is a very impersonal, unattractive way to choose a remedy but which nonetheless can be very effective. The successful use of computers, however, depends upon very accurate input and does not remove the need to check chosen remedies in a Materia Medica for the closest match to the patient.

It is important to remember Hahnemann's words on p. 38, in which he extols the virtues of peculiar symptoms by which to choose remedies. One should also recall the tremendous success Hahnemann and his disciples had with about 70 remedies and not be too ready to rush to new and exciting minor remedies. Those most commonly used are such because they fit, most often, the symptom picture of most conditions found.

In the veterinary application of Hahnemann's work and the work of repertory compilers we have to consider the likelihood that remedies might not always closely follow symptoms shown in humans when applied to animals. That is the first potential obstacle to the veterinary use of homoeopathy. As an illustration I cite the often excitatory effect of morphine derivatives in cats compared with no such effect in dogs, only the opposite occurring. One must, therefore, carefully study comparative toxicology and comparative pharmacology to select most accurately remedies of use in different species.

The second great obstacle in homoeopathic prescribing for animals and probably even greater than the first is the lack of mental symptoms gleaned from the patients in the history taking. These mental effects are ranked among Hahnemann's, and more especially his successors', most important pointers to prescribing (see paras. 210–211, Organon of Medicine). One can, however, extrapolate from behaviour and circumstance the most obvious ones in some cases and they can prove very useful. I take for example, grief at the loss of a mate or human companion, sexual frustration, anxiety, mental shock, fear, anger and sometimes even resentment at, for example, displacement from a human's affections by a new puppy.

The third great obstacle, caused by a limited ability to communicate with animals, is the paucity of symptoms of 'sensation' (subjective symptoms) that one can ascertain. For example is an arthritic pain tearing, burning, pulsating? Is an itch crawling, painful, biting, burning? These symptoms are obviously to be ranked among Hahnemann's symptoms peculiar to the disease and therefore of great importance in selecting a remedy. For instance, in the human case, I quote Kent's Repertory showing how such subjective symptoms affect choice of remedy: (p. 1081)

PAIN, FOOT, LIKE NAILS UNDER THE SKIN – *Rhus toxicodendron*

PAIN, FOOT, PULSATING – *Natrum carbonicum*

Clearly there is no hope of attaining this level of prescribing and therefore veterinary homoeopaths must lose some potential curative capability.

A fourth obstacle in translating the human repertories for animals is the presence of physiological and anatomical differences. How does one relate hair loss on the flanks of a dog to 'hair loss' in the human repertory? Can we correlate human menstruation with the blood flow at oestrus in the bitch? Does the front foot of an animal relate more to the human hand or the human foot in the repertory?

Homoeopathy in animals would be more widespread if such obstacles did not exist. For instance Kent lists 19 remedies useful in travel sickness.* How is one best to choose between them for animals? The remedies in Chapter 8 are the result of my attempts, and those of others, to select most commonly effective remedies from the many available to treat common ailments and disease syndromes, but the extent of possible deviation from that list (leading to incorrect choice of remedy) should now be clear.

In order to select a remedy for a case, and I firmly believe that a single remedy is the best ultimate solution even if not always attainable, one should decide at what level or levels to operate according to the relative chance of success. The possible levels of treatment are:

a) TREAT THE ROOT CAUSE or rather the inevitable *pathology* arising from that root cause (Pathological Level). A good example of an indication to choose this level of treatment is the case of road traffic injury where one would immediately use *Arnica* (because one can predict the pathology) whatever other

* Kent p. 509.

symptoms one may wish to treat either simultaneously or more usually subsequently. In the case of mental shock, also from whatever cause, one would leap to *Aconite.*

b) TREAT ACCORDING TO THE MENTAL SYMPTOMS. Where these are clearly discernible as mentioned on p. 41, it is a good idea to treat according to these first. They are very powerful movers in the cause of disease and can often be the crucial lead into a case representing the individuality of the patient (see also Chapter 12).

c) TREAT ACCORDING TO THE PRESENTING SYMPTOM. This is most commonly, but not always most effectively, the choice in cases coming into veterinary clinics. In this method of prescribing one uses the presenting sign as a cornerstone, made more precise by use of the modalities (see Chapters 9 and 17) and, very importantly, concomitant symptoms. The symptoms found in the case history, recorded under particulars, will prove a useful cross reference to choose between remedies. This is the method of shallow homoeopathy. Try to avoid relying too heavily on this method since it may end up only palliative in effect. It is only really useful in cases of simple, acute disease with an otherwise healthy constitution.

d) TREAT PREVIOUS UNDERLYING DISEASE (HISTORICAL). If a patient has experienced in the past (no matter how long ago) an over-ridingly powerful disease influence, such that the effects have never left completely, then it can sometimes be of no use to treat what you see, without first treating the previous disease. In this case the remedy to be selected is chosen as if the disease stimulus were still present at the time of examination (see Chapters 10, 11, 12, 14). The indication for this method is often betrayed by the phrase 'never well since . . . '. Such stimuli may be bereavement, injury, surgery, vaccination, etc. This principle can even apply when such diseases have occurred in the dam, especially if it was during the pregnancy which gave birth to this patient (see also Eugenics (q.v.)).

e) TREAT AT THE SO-CALLED CONSTITUTIONAL LEVEL. This is a post Hahnemann concept embodying the philosophy that most human individuals (and this can definitely be applied to animals depending upon one's aptitude to ascertain it) fall into distinct types, matched by a particular remedy usually from the list of very deep and wide acting remedies called the 'polycrests'. This typing is according to the programmed (hereditary, congenital and acquired) response to disease influence. If an animal clearly fits a 'type' portrayed under the description of remedies in materia medica, then application of this remedy will act upon the whole patient and produce a favourable tendency towards cure of *all* ailments experienced. It may not produce a full cure in many cases but will at least favourably affect the patient's response to another well-chosen remedy. Chronic disease invariably requires a constitutional prescription.

f) SPECIFIC LEVEL (see Chapter 11) and the

g) PREVENTIVE LEVEL (see Chapter 14) illustrate homoeopathy and isopathy in use against specific disease entities.

These usually involve the use of nosodes (q.v.). Care must be taken in the use of nosodes, particularly in the case of acute disease, for fear of serious aggravation with dangerous consequences.

h) FACILITATIVE/REGULATORY/DETOXIFYING prescribing exploits the ability of potentised substances to modify, modulate or regulate the body's absorptive, metabolic and excretory processes with respect to that substance. One can, for example, use potentised calcium salts to regulate calcium metabolism, potentised hormones to regulate hormone balance (p. 115) potentised minerals to facilitate absorption of those minerals or potentised toxins to speed elimination of those specific toxins.*

i) ORGAN SPECIFIC PRESCRIBING utilises the fact that certain remedies have an affinity for certain organs or tissues (e.g. *Nux vomica* for the liver or *Hypericum* for nerve tissue) and can act as a useful adjunct to therapy.

Examples of the above levels of prescribing can be found in Chapter 16. Taking all these factors into consideration shows the limitations imposed by strictly adhering to guidelines shown in

---

* N.B. *Sulphur* and *Nux vomica*, among other remedies, can serve as 'cleaning' or detoxifying remedies. The French refer to *drénage* and some prescribers follow a strict 'drainage' routine.

Chapters 8–14. One must be prepared to deviate from the 'ready reckoner' type of prescribing in order to be reasonably successful.

If a remedy fails to fit very well or if two or three remedies could be chosen on seemingly equal merits, should one try to stick to one remedy, as Hahnemann and many since him maintain, or should one use two or three compatible remedies? One should, at all times, try to find one correct remedy because in this way, when a case is difficult, one is forced to delve deeper into both the patient and the books and this is a useful exercise. It also, in my opinion, provides the best ultimate cure. If, however, one feels a cure depends upon a rapid selection of a remedy it should do no harm to the case to use two or three remedies. All one loses is the depth and power of the single remedy and the knowledge of which remedy worked, so an opportunity for experience is lost. (There is a further hazard of incompatibility of remedies but this is difficult to evaluate.)* The use of manufactured compound remedies (usually 5 or more homoeopathic remedies made into a single product) is common in some countries and such preparations have found their way into the UK. They are part of the modern trend of commercialism and are often marketed with specific disease syndromes indicated. This method of prescribing can be effective in some cases but will never achieve the depth of cure of a single correct remedy and will tend to slow or prevent the prescriber's personal development in homoeopathy. The fact that such combinations can also serve to 'confuse' the vital force may result in dangerous confusion of the case and ultimate failure to cure. A further discussion of this occurs in the next chapter in relation to potency. One cannot, in the end, rule out the part played by intuition (part of our valuable sixth sense) in selecting a level of prescribing or in choosing the key symptoms upon which to prescribe a homoeopathic remedy.

* I have been asked many times to put into words my ideas on combination of different levels of prescribing. In order to achieve rapid results I combine on occasions, say, the 'constitutional' approach with, say, the 'presenting symptom' approach. This can have the added advantage, if the patient is able to respond, of stimulating the vital force at more than one level at once. This would not be justifiable in strictly hahnemannian terms but does produce some very worthwhile results. One can use more than two levels at the same time. I have presented a schematic approach to this problem in my new book 'The Homoeopathic Treatment of Beef and Dairy Cattle' in Chapter 5. In summary, however, I believe overuse of multiple remedies will result in a 'confused' case and may even so distort the vital force as to amount to a dangerous procedure (see pp. 43, 53, 156/157).

CHAPTER 6

Putting Principles into Practice 3
*Managing the Case**

Having decided upon the level of treatment to be employed and having chosen carefully that remedy which will best serve the case, there are still further decisions to be made:

By what route should the remedy be applied?
What physical form of the remedy should be used?
What potency should be selected?
What frequency of dosing should be set?
For how long should the dose be given (duration)?
When should the effect be checked?
How should the effect of a correct remedy/close remedy/wrong remedy/wrong potency be assessed?

I think it is worth discussing all these questions at length, although this does not mean I am claiming any great knowledge on these difficult points.

ROUTE OF ADMINISTRATION

The choice must be tailored to suit the conditions to be treated. For example where the whole system is affected by the condition or the condition is caused by an internal derangement then, because the whole body is involved, the whole body must be treated. In this instance, go for an oral or parenteral treatment (that is by mouth or

* See also p. 115

injection) to achieve the desired effect. The condition may, at the same time, demand a topical treatment of superficial lesions but Hahnemann does draw attention to potential problems with topical treatments in chronic cases. Where a lesion is considered to be purely of local significance e.g. an abrasion or cut, topical treatment may be all that is required but sometimes oral treatment in addition may be beneficial and may hasten healing.

Injections are more often used in the farm application than in the small animal surgery for the reason that it is not easily practical to give a cow pills several times daily. Injections appear to be effective despite some prescribers' misgivings. In the small animal clinic however, the very experience that most animals fear about conventional veterinary medicine is the injections, so it is a great advantage for homoeopathy that medicines are given orally for dogs and cats.

Water medication is very useful in the farm animal context and in the cage-bird or cage-pet situation (see Chapter 11). There is less control over frequency by this method but it avoids the need to handle fragile and fearful pet animals and free-roaming farm livestock. It is also makes it possible to treat a whole group of animals with a single administration.

PHYSICAL FORM OF REMEDY

The choice of form of preparation in which a remedy is prescribed is in part personal and in part governed by the same considerations as above. Pillules, tablets and powders are ideal for oral administration, although my personal preference is for pillules. Lotions, tinctures, creams and ointments are ideal for the topical situation. Tinctures suit water administration but pills will also serve in the water container for a cage bird or cage mammal, if a tincture in a required remedy is not available. Tinctures can be used orally undiluted but may be rejected, especially by cats, on account of their alcohol content. They must always be diluted before topical use, especially on tender surfaces e.g. eyes, mucous membranes or sores and wounds. Two or three drops in an eggcupful of water is sufficient strength for such application.

POTENCY

Whenever the subject of potency is raised some people become excited and some even frightened. The tendency is to have very fixed opinions on the subject or to be totally overawed by it. I hope this section will help to unravel some of the mysteries. It would appear to be agreed by most that, as the potency increases, so does the depth and duration of action. What is lost in this process is breadth of action. High potencies are considered for the purpose of this text to be above **12c**, low potencies below **6c**. **6c** to **12c** seems to be a 'watershed' (see p. 13 and Appendix 3).

If one is sure of a remedy for a case one can confidently use a high potency and be sure of its effect. If one is not so sure of the remedy the potency should be kept lower, giving a wider spread of action (see figs. 2–6)

A fertile imagination is needed to gain a graphic concept of the workings of a homoeopathic remedy against disease. Firstly assume there is a curative 'window' through which the remedy must pass to effect a cure. Imagine, then, a disease entity with several symptom sites (□) and a disease centre: (✕):

Figs. 2 and 3

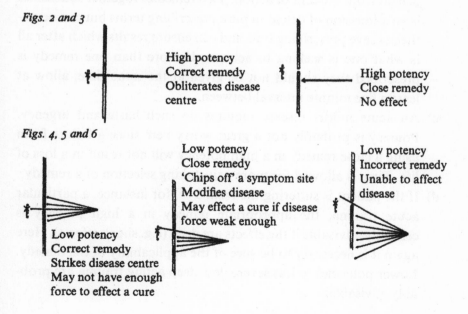

High potency
Correct remedy
Obliterates disease
centre

High potency
Close remedy
No effect

Figs. 4, 5 and 6

Low potency
Close remedy
'Chips off' a symptom site
Modifies disease
May effect a cure if disease
force weak enough

Low potency
Incorrect remedy
Unable to affect
disease

Low potency
Correct remedy
Strikes disease centre
May not have enough
force to effect a cure

The next step when choosing a potency is to consider the patient itself and its disease.

a) Is it a chronic disease?
b) Is it an acute dramatic disease?
c) Is it an acute milder disease?
d) Is it the result of a particular agency e.g. trauma?
e) Could a constitutional remedy be used?
f) Is the condition brought about by an overriding mental condition?
g) Is the patient still suffering the effects of a previous illness?

Running through these questions in order:

a) A chronic disease by definition has been about a long time and gone deep and will most likely take a while to recede. If you are sure of the remedy, a high potency is valuable in order to obtain the depth of cure required. I use **30c** and above. Often I have found the need to increase potency after a short period on **30**, since the effectiveness seems to wane in some cases, probably as a result of all the curative power of that potency having been utilised.

b) An acute and dramatic disease will brook no delay in activity. Unless absolutely certain of a remedy use **6c** or lower in order to benefit from breadth of action. Two remedies together sometimes is an admission of defeat in pure prescribing terms but can nevertheless save prescribing time and can ensure results which after all is what one is seeking to achieve. If more than one remedy is prescribed they should not be given at the same time; allow at least a five minute interval between.

c) An acute milder disease requires no such haste and urgency. Potency is probably not a great worry here since a failure from using a close remedy in a high potency will not result in a loss of life. Time is allowed for more painstaking selection of a remedy.

d) If the patient is suffering the results of, for instance, a particular acute trauma, the appropriate remedy in a high potency is certainly advisable if the effects are deep (e.g. shock effects). Here again it is necessary to be sure of the applicability of the remedy. Lower potencies in less severe, less deep acting trauma are probably advisable.

e) If a constitutional remedy is used, one is presumably sure of that remedy or the indication for the remedy would not have been felt. Since the animal's constitution is deep go for high potency.

f) In the case of mental conditions (e.g. bereavement) higher potencies are a good idea but one needs to be sure of the remedy, otherwise go for low.

g) If a previous illness is suspected of still causing trouble it must be eliminated by a deep acting remedy, that is, in a high potency (see p. 13).

As a general guide, I suggest in summary that a higher potency may be used in cases where the vitality (vital force) is strong and vibrant, in acute disease, where lower potencies have failed to elicit a full response and in cases in which the prescriber is sure of the remedy. I suggest that a high potency should not be used in the very old, in ailing cancer cases, in acute disease when the vitality is struck very low or in any other case in which the vital force is considered to be very weak or in mortal danger.

In all cases, if a remedy is needed rapidly and you have it on the shelf, even if only in the potency least suited in your opinion to the case, use the potency you have to hand. That must be better than not using it at all. It must however be remembered that many remedies appear to have a clearly different effect according to potency, that is they are regulatory in their effect or tend more obviously to display 'biphasic' activity. Some examples are:

Hepar sulph.   low potency provokes suppuration,
                high potency aborts suppuration.

Merc. sol.   Similarly

Folliculinum   low potency arouses female activity,
                7c regulates female activity,
                12c and above restrains female activity.

Urtica urens   low potency depresses milk flow,
                high potency stimulates milk flow.

Salvia   low potency reduces perspiration,
                high potency stimulates perspiration.

Thyroidinum   low potency stimulates the thyroid gland,
                high potency suppresses its activity (p. 115)

FREQUENCY

Hahnemann always suggested not giving a second dose until the first had worn off. In the case of easily measurable responses this principle should be followed. Chronic diseases demand a less frequent repetition than acute conditions where, in really acute severe cases, doses can even be given every ten minutes. This is true even in the higher potencies. Once the effect is observed doses can be given less frequently according to effect. In chronic conditions, administration once or twice daily for a few days and then waiting until an effect is noticed is a very useful guideline. (See also prevention of disease, Chapter 14.)

DURATION

The dose of a confidently selected remedy should be kept up until the effect is seen. After this one should dose 'to effect', the intervals sometimes becoming so long as to constitute a cessation of treatment. The answer to the question 'how long?' is therefore unanswerable in specific time units. Treatment for chronic conditions can be expected to extend over weeks or even months in extreme cases but acute conditions should demand no more than two or three days in the main.

FOLLOW UP VISITS

How soon should a case be checked for response? A veterinarian must decide at what interval he should ask to see the patient again. The main reason to see the patient again is to assess effectiveness of the remedy, therefore there is again the distinction between acute and chronic conditions. As a rough guide it seems practical to say that acute severe cases should report on the same day, acute milder cases should report on the following day but chronic cases according to the expected progress rate, at one or two weekly intervals or even longer intervals in some cases. In skin cases in particular, an interval of three weeks is often a good guide.

ASSESSMENT

When a patient returns to the surgery an assessment of progress must be made in order to ascertain whether, at the first attempt:*

the correct remedy at the correct potency was chosen,
the correct remedy but wrong potency was chosen,
a close remedy was chosen,
the wrong frequency was chosen,
the wrong duration was chosen.

After the chosen interval on a correct remedy at the correct potency one can see:

a) In the case of a chronic condition, with or without an improvement in the obvious symptoms, a distinct improvement in the well-being of the patient as a whole. Continue treatment, according to frequency and duration principles (p. 50).

b) In the case of a chronic condition, a failure to alter the presenting complaint along with a disturbing recurrence of a previous complaint (recapitulation of the earlier stages of chronic disease) which may at the time have been considered unrelated to the present complaint. Continue treatment as above.

c) The cure can, again in a chronic condition, work from within outwards so that deeper troubles (e.g. heart, digestive, mental) clear up before, say, a skin complaint. Continue treatment as above.

d) A complete cure or good progress along that route can occur in a very short time. Only continue treatment if necessary.

e) It is possible to have selected correctly and fail to achieve any result whatsoever. In this case it is possible that one has missed, in the earlier history taking, the significance of an overriding effect of an earlier disease not completely cured. Canine Parvovirus or Feline Enteritis, Leptospiral Jaundice, difficult pregnancy, various mental considerations can all (with many other conditions) leave their mark. The correct nosode or similium should be applied

---

* For the purpose of this section I am assuming no conventional drug (suppressive) factors are present. These can lead to even greater complexities as the drug effects wear off upon stopping drug intake.

without delay (see p. 129 et seq. and p. 42 (d)). External influences, such as diet or action of chemicals, may also limit the effect of the correct homoeopathic remedy and provide an obstacle to recovery. These must be checked and corrected where necessary.

There are several indications of a correct remedy in the wrong potency having been chosen:

a) An apparent worsening of the disease (aggravation). The treatment should be discontinued forthwith to test if this is the case. If so the effect will be temporary and a cure can often ensue. Continue treatment later with a higher potency if the condition does not resolve fully. Rarely a lower potency may be needed.

b) Inadequate depth of effect with no different symptoms emerging may indicate a remedy in too low a potency.

c) Rarely, a local pathological condition will fail to respond to too high a potency, where it seems that the remedy runs on too high a plane for the disease presented. It can be analogous to shooting over the enemy's head. If sure of the remedy, lower the potency.

In all cases of a correct remedy having been chosen, there should be no alteration in nature of symptoms shown.

An incorrect remedy that is very close can produce a change in symptoms (see figs. 2–6, p. 47) if the potency is low enough. Go back to square one and take account of the new symptoms in order to choose the correct remedy. Often it is a closely related remedy that is required, such as prescribed *Mercurius corr.* needing, instead, *Mercurius sol.*

A wrong remedy produces no effect if it is not close enough or not in low enough potency (see figs. 2–6, p. 47). Alternatively, there can be a basic alteration in nature of symptoms. Go back to the history notes to find the error in prescribing, remembering especially the possible adverse influence of previous disease, which has been suppressed, against an apparently correct remedy (see p. 42 (d)). Retake the case too, in order to update your records fully.

Rarely a remedy can be correct, produce benefit and then fail. A second remedy can then be needed and eventually an alternation of the two may be required. *Rhus tox.* and *Bryonia* commonly show this alternating relationship, where the modalities of a rheumatic condition alternate between those of these two remedies.

If doses are given too frequently or for too long a great confusion can arise. At first the case may improve but then it can relapse to varying degrees. This can be a result of having carried out a 'proving' (that is producing the symptoms of the remedy, as did Hahnemann in his very first tests). The confusion then confronting the prescriber is:

a) Is the remedy wrong; the change in the disease being a coincidental improvement then relapse?

b) Is a correct remedy prescribed wrongly, so producing a proving?

To unravel this, all one can do is cease treatment immediately and observe results. Usually it is a proving and the symptoms will rapidly subside. I think it is important that no prescription should be refilled without the knowledge of the prescribing veterinarian, in order to prevent unwitting over treatment* (see also pp. 43/44, 155/156).

Whereas it is often said that there are no side effects of homoeopathic treatment some of the aforementioned sequelae could be misread as such. They are clearly not side effects in the true sense of the word, merely extraneous effects of the primary purpose, nor do they last. An open mind is essential, not only before prescribing but, as the foregoing points demonstrate, after prescribing too. The sequelae of the treatment must be read with care and acted upon correctly in order to achieve the deep and lasting cure for which one strives.

---

* We are not discussing here the amount given at any one time. This factor appears to be unimportant. As long as the organism is *introduced* to the potentised remedy there is no need to worry about body size, etc. The dose appears to be energetic in nature and therefore not dependent upon actual *quantity* of medicine given.

CHAPTER 7

Putting Principles into Practice 4
Care of the Remedies

Very little is understood of the real nature of homoeopathic remedies in potency. There is still no accepted reliable method of measuring their quality and this reason alone is enough to suggest that it is sensible only to acquire them from reputable sources. Having acquired them it is of major importance to look after them very carefully to ensure that their efficacy is not lost during their potentially very long life. This applies as well to their storage in a veterinary clinic as to that in the home.

The nature of the remedy appears to be a form of energy pattern harnessed from the original substance during the potentising process. This pattern is then imprinted upon the carrier whether it be a solvent in liquid remedies or a powder or tablet in the use of solid preparations. Thus, although all conventionally measurable traces of the original substance are lost, and with them the power to produce side effects, the curative power is enhanced and trapped in what must be a relatively labile form.

It is not necessary to go to the lengths of air-conditioned storage, special containers and so forth but it is essential to be reasonably careful to choose a storage place for them which allows them to remain in a fairly constant environment. This environment should be free from excessive damp, cold or heat, free from direct sunlight and clear of all very strong smelling substances.

Camphor preparations, in homoeopathic potency or mother tinctures, should be stored separately. Containers should be glass but, although there is talk of long term damage to a remedy by storage in plastic, there appears to be no short-term deleterious effect. Permeable products such as paper or cardboard should not be used since they are too subject to influence from the environment.

The pills should not be handled except when actually administering the remedy to the patient, any pills that have been handled should not be returned to the bottle. Pills may conveniently be dispensed into the bottle cap prior to dosing and, if the patient allows, be tossed from the cap directly into the mouth. This method removes the need for handling at all, which can reduce or damage the remedy's efficacy. The bottles of two remedies should not be opened at the same time, and there should be at least a five minute interval between giving doses of different remedies. The remedies should not be given with food.

One day much of this book may be rendered obsolete and especially this chapter, as research (actively proceeding at present) unfolds more of the nature of remedies and their mode of action. Many beliefs passed on in these pages may seem strange when it is known what 'potency' really is and it can be measured. Then it will be possible to ascertain exactly what does and does not affect it. Until that day, however, I think it is important to adhere to the above advice in order to ensure the maximum efficacy and long shelf 'life' of purchased remedies.

CHAPTER 8

Symptoms of Disease with some Recommended Treatments

This chapter is designed around the basic layout of Kent's Repertory for the body systems and should fit well with the history taking (Particulars section) see Chapter 4. Symptoms of the mind (Mentals), appearing first in most repertories as a very important prescribing factor in human medicine, will be dealt with on their own later (Chapter 12), since there has not yet been devised a way of giving it priority in all cases of animal disease. I must reiterate that this chapter should not be used as a 'bible' of veterinary homoeopathy in small animals but as a guide in methodology and as an insight into some very useful remedies. Please do be sure to read a wider selection of books than this one alone (see bibliography). Please also be encouraged to read the chapters on principles before using this chapter. The use of these remedies is bound to be more successful if a wider understanding of homoeopathy is attained prior to attempting its practice. Please also adhere to good nursing and dietary principles (additional notes p. 115).

The symptoms to be discussed will appear under the following headings in the order given:

Head and Face, Eyes, Ears, Nose, Mouth, Digestive System, Urinary System, Male Sexual System, Female Sexual System (including Breeding), Respiratory System, Heart, Circulatory and Blood System, Lymphatic System, Locomotor System, Skin, Nervous System, Endocrines.

Some variation is shown from Kent and Boericke for which I make no apology. The needs of the veterinarian are different from those of the physician. I suggest that the notes from the clinical examination follow the above order for convenience.

Many apparent opportunities for expansion, inclusion of further symptoms and remedies etc., will appear to the observant reader but I felt that, in compiling this chapter, too full a discussion would lead to loss of clarity and direction. It is not intended to be a total veterinary manual. A greater attempt in this direction could be made in a future volume on all species. If no mention is made of species please assume the comments apply to all species. Exceptions will be highlighted.

When a remedy is given under a particular disease or symptom it is very likely to be useful if one can match the properties of the remedy shown in Chapter 17 with other concomitant symptoms in the patient. Remedies fitting the generalities of the case can always be used if indicated in addition to those described (see p. 42). Constitutional prescribing is of especial importance in chronic disease.

Serious conditions require veterinary help.

HEAD AND FACE

One must distinguish between disease of the bones of head and face and disease of the accompanying soft tissues (muscles, skin, etc.). For diseases of injury refer to appropriate sections on this subject (p. 123). For injury to the brain and disease of the brain see Nervous System.

Pathology Encountered in the Head and Facial Area

a) BONY LUMPS (Exostoses) or DEFORMITIES:
   These can occur anywhere on the head for unknown reasons or as a result of previous injury. Remedies powerfully effective in this field are:

Forehead, upper jaw and nasal area	*Aurum met.*
Lower jaw with degenerative changes	*Calc. fluor.*
Especially lower jaw with lymph nodes swollen (can include cranium and upper jaw)	*Hekla lava.*

This latter pattern is seen especially in Craniomandibular Osteopathy in the West Highland White Terrier. Also of use in this condition are *Pituitary Extracts* or *Thyroid* in potency.

With tooth involvement especially upper jaw and under eyes, putrid breath, profuse saliva, facial deformity, swollen lymph nodes and contracture of masticatory muscles	*Mercurius sol.*

The picture of **Malar abscess** fits this general picture wherein the conventional course of action is extraction of the offending tooth. Homoeopathy is still a very useful adjunct to this treatment.

Swelling and necrosis of the jaw bone with puffy eyelids etc.	*Phosphorus*
Discrete swelling on (especially) lower jaw	*Kali iod.*
Swelling and atrophy of turbinates with consequent distortion of the nose in young animals	*Lemna minor*

b) SOFT TISSUES:

Allergy shows frequently in the facial area as an urticarial swelling of the eyelids, and possibly entire face. Apart from ascertaining the cause if possible, treat according to symptoms (possibly with *Galphimia glauca* in low potency as a general 'antiallergic' remedy).

With irritation (worse for cold)	*Urtica urens*
Oedema and pain (worse for heat)	*Apis mel.*
Upper eyelids especially	*Kali carb.*
Cheeks, lips, crusted eyes, stopped up nose	*Bovista*
Swollen upper and lower eyelids	*Phosphorus*

These remedies are only suggestions with general guiding symptoms provided. See also Conjunctivitis (p. 60) and Eyelids (p. 61). Generally this problem is seen in dogs but cats can sometimes show it especially in reaction to an antibiotic.

Cellulitis in a cat's face following a cat bite should not be confused with this condition (use *Hepar sulph.*). Where incomplete abscessation or recurring suppuration from an old wound occurs use *Silica*.

Myositis (inflammation of the muscle) generally only occurs in one specific condition of unknown aetiology but injury may be involved – Temporal Myositis (also called Eosinophilic Myositis or Atrophic Myositis). It is usually seen in large breeds of dog. The muscles over the head and around the throat become inflamed, painful and swollen and in more advanced cases shrink (contracture). Eating and swallowing become increasingly difficult and the patient may become vicious as a result of pain and distress. Voice change, locked jaw and changed facial expression can occur (cf. Tetanus). This picture is beautifully matched by *Cedron*. As a nerve may be involved, cure is not necessarily assured. Nursing assumes vital importance. Other remedies which can be of use are: *Aconite*, *Arnica*, *Gelsemium* and *Hypericum*. Use *Mercurius sol.* where contracture is noticeable. *Kali iod*, may also be of use. Acupuncture is also helpful

Opisthotonus is a symptom in which the head is drawn back over the neck and shoulders. The forelimbs are usually extended see Tetanus p. 130 and Nervous System p. 111.

Furunculosis affects the nose area, chin and upper jaw mostly. There is usually a deep infection with Staphylococcus and often follicular mange. Use: *Staphylococcus nosode*, *Silica*, *Hepar sulph.* Constitutional treatment is also important. Topical mange treatment may be used if absolutely necessary but the author is worried about the safety and wisdom of some of the chemicals used, esp. organophosphorus compounds (see also Skin p. 106 and Eyelids p. 61).

Head Gland Disease. This is a very serious extension of the above problem, involving the whole head in some cases and the lymph glands of the head and neck. It responds well to homoeopathy, especially if caught in the early stages and remedies are similar to the above. However, the author advises veterinary help, since the condition can worsen rapidly and become out of control if the incorrect remedy is chosen.

Rodent ulcer see Mouth and Skin.

EYES

Eye conditions constitute one of the more spectacular spheres of action for homoeopathy. Conventional medicine finds the eyes difficult to treat but careful selection of the correct homoeopathic remedy can achieve amazing results. Treatment of eyes is best left to the veterinarian, since close examination of the eye is essential and consequences of failure are serious.

Disorders of Eye Movement are dealt with under Nervous System p. III.

All superficial inflammation of the eye and eye area can be helped by *Calendula* lotion, or tincture diluted. Also *Euphrasia* eye lotion is a very useful preparation where symptoms indicate and is a general aid to healing of the eye and associated tissues.

Injury to eye and eye area is dealt with under Injury p. 123. Check for foreign body.

Conjunctivitis. A great number of remedies act on the conjunctiva but only the most useful ones will be discussed here:

Intensely red or pink conjunctiva profuse micropurulent discharge, granular conjunctivitis, with or without clouding of the cornea and photophobia (abdominal symptoms may accompany)	*Argent. nit.*
Conjunctivitis acquired by travelling with head out of car window or aggravated by cold, dry wind, eyes water profusely and patient rubs them	*Euphrasia*
Profuse lachrymation, dilated pupils, photophobia, also aggravated by cold winds	*Aconite*
After removal of foreign bodies or after operations	*Aconite*
Worse at night and worse for heat	*Sulphur*
Agglutination, photophobia, burning corrosive tears, eyes dull and sunken	*Arsen. alb.*
Bland tears, sensitive to light	*Allium cepa*
Sensitive to light, comes and goes, creamy pus, desire to rub, worse for wind	*Pulsatilla*

With photophobia, cloudy cornea, especially older dog, yellow sclera, no inflammation	*Conium mac.*
Lids red and inflamed, burning discharges, leaving white flakes	*Sanicula*
Granular, purulent, spreads down face	*Jequirity* (*Arbrus precatorius*)
Watery and itchy, worse in open air and after exercise	*Sabadilla*
With sore cheeks, itchiness, agglutination, dilated pupil, suppuration	*Ledum*
Photophobia, very injected sclera, corneal ulcer, blepharospasm	*Merc. sol.*
Worse photophobia, very constricted pupil	*Merc. cor.*
Red margins of lids, inflammation from foreign body, cold air aggravates, quivering lids, dilated pupils, morning agglutination	*Calc. carb.*
Spasm of lids, red, corrosive tears, usually lateral canthus	*Natrum mur.*
Not affected by light, insensible, cloudy	*Lycopodium*
Photophobia, rubbing, profuse lachrymation, nose waters	*Cobaltum*
From entropion or trichiasis	*Borax*
Photophobia, enlarged meibomian glands, purulent	*Rhus tox.*
Ropy pus, yellowish, itching oedema, no pain or photophobia	*Kali bich.*

Nosodes of Distemper or Cat 'flu, if these viruses are or have been involved, can prove very useful (or even vital) adjuncts to treatment by the appropriate similium.

Eyelids

Growths. Conventionally these are removed but it is well worth trying homoeopathic treatment first to try to prevent this eventuality. Useful remedies are:

Kali iod., *Conium* (old dog syndrome), *Staphisagria* (hard lumps in margins) and especially *Thuja*.

Inflammation. Primarily consider *Rhus tox.*, if other mucocutaneous junctions involved consider *Nitric acid*. Most of the conjunctivitis remedies can apply here according to the similia principle (use the preceding pages as a guide). If the lids are red and painful and granulated in appearance and there is swelling of the face consider *Cinnabaris*, see also Furunculosis p. 59.

Entropion. *Borax* is the prime remedy here and may avert surgery. It is a long term treatment.

If gross conjunctivitis with blephoraspasm	*Natrum mur.*
Where inflammation of lids has caused swelling leading to inturned eyelids	*Tellurium*

Fissures in Eyelids. *Graphites* or *Petroleum* are indicated but other skin signs usually guide one to the correct remedy.

Trichiasis and Dystichiasis (misplaced, or extra eyelashes). *Borax* is worth trying but repeated plucking is also advisable, since they are so able to damage the eye.

Lachrymal Duct and Glands

Meibomian Glands in the margins of the lids can become inflamed. This is almost impossible to distinguish from inflammation of the eyelid and conjunctiva.

The same remedies apply according to symptoms shown, especially:	*Rhus tox.*
If intolerance of milk is involved	*Aethusa*

Lachrymal Duct Blockage usually a chronic sequel of feline viral respiratory infections. Rarely blocked in dogs. May also be sequel of injury.

Argentum met., *Calc. carb.*, *Pulsatilla*, *Silica*, *Symphytum* according to symptoms.

Lachrymal Gland Inflamed – *Hepar sulph.*, *Iodum* (acute), *Pulsatilla*, *Silica* according to symptoms.

Affections of Lachrymal Puncta (opening in lower lid) – *Cinnabaris*.

If the Lachrymal Gland ceases to function this leads to the serious condition of Keratitis Sicca, 'Dry Eye'. This affects especially West Highland White Terriers and aetiology is not known. False tears are an essential immediate first aid to prevent damage to the cornea. To prevent surgery being necessary try *Zincum met.*, *Veratrum alb.*, or *Senega*, with a constitutional remedy (see case history Chapter 16).

The Cornea

This is the bright clear front of the eyeball through which light passes to the lens. Its clarity is upset by any damage or change in the fluid balance system, which is maintained by evaporation from the front surface and replenishment from the chamber behind. There are no blood vessels in the normal cornea.

Ulceration, pigmentation, vascularisation, cloudiness, granular appearance and rupture are all possible conditions to be observed. All may be successfully resolved if correctly treated homoeopathically and if treatment is started in good time. Management of these conditions represents one of the special wonders of homoeopathy. The eye, despite its fragile appearance, has the most wonderful powers of recovery if correctly encouraged. All forms of surgery for the cornea should be avoidable if one obtains a favourable response to treatment.

Blueing of the Cornea is an occasional side effect of Hepatitis vaccination in the dog. The *Hepatitis nosode* is useful.

Cloudiness: This can be a sign of inflammation of the cornea (keratitis) or a part of a general ageing process.

Keratitis often in conjunction with conjunctivitis; many remedies serve both.

Cloudy, inflamed conjunctiva, with purulent
discharge   *Argentum nit.*

Pearly white conjunctiva, some glaucoma (swollen eye from internal pressure)	*Phosphorus*
Showing internal ill health, dull eye, fails to respond to light, nose stopped up, fan like movement of nostrils, liver symptoms	*Lycopodium*
Chronic dilation of pupils, cataract, usually stocky, possibly flabby constitution	*Calc. carb.*
No pain or photophobia	*Kali bich.*
Very photophobic	*Merc. cor.*
With very dilated pupil, some glaucoma	*Belladonna*
Cornea like ground glass, ophthalmia present, early ulcer, night aggravation	*Sulphur*

Opacity:

Usually with cataract	*Calc. fluor.*
With cataract	*Causticum*
With purulent conjunctivitis	*Argent. nit.*
Water all the time, conjunctivitis, blueing	*Euphrasia*
With sneezing coryza	*Naphthalinum*

Cineraria eye lotion is very useful, especially after injury (long term treatment). *Silica* removes scars after ulceration, injury, surgery etc. (long term treatment).

Both cloudiness and opacity can result from Keratitis Sicca (see p. 63). If a result of ageing, consider *Conium*.

Corneal Ulceration: In this condition the outer membrane of the cornea is lost in one area as a result of infection, inflammation or damage. More layers may become affected and eventually rupture is possible (see sequelae). Surgery should be avoidable in all cases. The condition is often accompanied by great photophobia (see p. 192).

Purulent discharge, red conjunctiva, closes eye, cornea clouds almost to the point of being opaque, photophobia in warm room	*Argent. nit.*

Anyone who has seen what a 'styptic pencil' can do to the front of the eye will know what *Argent. nit.* can cure.

Indolent ulcer in a fat subject (usually), with
or without cataract, usually aged dog   *Calc. carb.*
Watery eye, frequent blinking, swollen lids,
sticky mucus on cornea, photophobia,
especially in daylight, corneal opacity or
blueness   *Euphrasia*
Swollen lids, ropy mucus, very little pain, deep
ulceration, conjunctivitis   *Kali bich.*
A truly wonderful remedy in the case of great
photophobia, fear of the eye being touched, no
pupil movement, deep ulceration (other mercurial
signs are usually present e.g. thirst with wet
mouth, smelly breath)   *Merc. cor.*
A very similar remedy with less photophobia and
more chronicity   *Merc. sol.*
Also of use in cases of great photophobia   *Conium*
In cases where suppurative processes have
started or with pus in the eye itself too
(hypopion). This occurs especially after cat claw
injuries to the eye   *Hepar sulph.*

Injury:
Puncture   *Ledum*
Laceration   *Staphisagria*

Sequelae
Perforation giving rise to Keratocoele or Staphyloma (swellings on the
front of the eye):

In early stages to reduce swelling   *Apis mel.*
To complete healing   *Merc. sol.*

Vascularisation and Pigmentation: *Merc. sol.* is a very effective long
term treatment, but early effects are immediately obvious.
If great photophobia   *Aurum met.*

Opaque scars: Long term treatment   *Silica*

{65}

Lens

Cataract, is an opacity of the lens, not always possible to clear but *Cineraria* eye lotion, in the long term, can help clear or slow the condition. Also use:–

Cloudy lens	*Sulphur*
Aged dog and from injury	*Conium*
Incipient cataract	*Nat. mur.*
Fat, indigestion, ageing	*Calc. carb.*
Degeneration with age	*Phosphorus*
Degeneration after eye surgery	*Senega*
Dry or opaque, usually sneezing coryza	*Naphthalinum*

Also *Silica 30* as long term treatment may help and consider *Calc. fluor.* but do not repeat too often.

Pupil

The pupil of the eye is designed to open and close in response to dark and light respectively. When this fails to happen it is a symptom to be noted. It is either dilated or contracted.

PUPIL DILATED:
Argent. nit.,
*Belladonna,
Calc. carb. (ageing),
Conium (injury or ageing),
Gelsemium,
Glonoinium (especially useful in heat stroke),
Hyoscyamus,
Spigelia (eye, heart, nervous system remedy),
Stramonium.

Thus, when concomitant symptoms are correct for any of these remedies (or others), they may be used with confidence.
Glaucoma can occur with pupil dilation (see p. 67).
Also remember *Symphytum* if orbital area is damaged by trauma, *Helleborus* if concussion.

Key Gaskell Syndrome in cats, a newly discovered syndrome,* may be helped most satisfactorily in its early stages by *Belladonna, Calc. carb., Hyoscyamus, Stramonium* or *Wyethia* (dilated pupils are a major symptom). *Gelsemium* can also play a part. See separate section on p. 134.

PUPIL CONTRACTED: In cases of Ophthalmitis (q.v.), that is, inflammation of whole eye, contracted pupil can lead to, or is a result of, pain. In cases of pupilloconstriction consider:

With nervous cause	*Opium, Phyostigmine.*
With Ophthalmitis	*Rhus tox.*
Usually with conjunctivitis	*Thuja.*

Contracted pupil may also be a symptom of lead poisoning. Use *Plumbum met.* with the similium. It is important both to relieve the poisoning and to remove the source.

Again there are a great many more remedies which can help contracted pupils. Concomitant symptoms must be the guide to selection.

Arnica can be used with dilated or contracted pupils, if as a result of injury to brain or head. Similarly *Helleborus,* although this usually suits a dilated pupil, with eyes turned upwards.

Eyeball

Glaucoma is a condition of the eyeball where the pressure within is so great as to make the eye swell, thus damaging its internal structures including the optic nerve. Since the angle of drainage in the anterior chamber is opened by pupillo-constriction a dilated pupil is not a desirable symptom (see Pupils dilated). Acupuncture helps.

GLAUCOMA REMEDIES:

Early stage of fever	*Aconite*
With pupil dilation and other concomitant signs	*Belladonna*
With ophthalmitis	*Phosphorus*

Also *Gelsemium* and *Spigelia*. Again select a remedy according to concomitants.

* At time of 1st Edition, but now rarely seen (also called Feline Dysautonomia).

Ophthalmitis (total, deep inflammation of the eye). This is a very painful condition. The pupil is usually constricted in response to the pain which, because of tension in the muscle of the pupil, increases the pain; a vicious circle.

Remedies most likely to help in this condition:

with pupillo constriction, purulent discharge, rheumatics	*Rhus tox.
With pupil dilation	Belladonna
	*Phosphorus
In early stages	Aconite
If clouding in the eye	Euphrasia
If blood in the eye	Hamamelis
With catarrhal inflammation	Kali bich.
If pus present (use high potency)	Hepar sulph.
Redness of whole eye	Cinnabaris

Quick action is necessary to avoid permanent damage to the sensitive eye structures.

Use *Symphytum* if you suspect injury to the eyeball by a blow from a blunt instrument.

Orbital Area. Physical damage to the area is potentially serious and *Symphytum* seems to have an uncanny effect on any injury caused by a blow from a blunt object e.g. dog kicked by a horse. *Hamamelis* and *Arnica* are also useful, *Hamamelis* especially where there is bleeding into the eye. *Conium* has its special sphere of action affecting surgical injury to this area and to the eye.

Other useful remedies are:

Puncture wound to the eye	Ledum
Cellulitis	Rhus tox.
Oedematous swelling	Apis mel.
Growths or periostitis	Kali iod.

A rare sequel to a blow on the head is **detached retina**.

Gelsemium is favoured here although the author has no experience of this. *Naphthalinum* is also indicated.

Epiphora (overflow of tears) see blocked Lachrymal duct, p. 62 and Influenza p. 132. Consider also:

Alium cepa, Cobaltum, Euphrasia, Sabadilla.

Everyone has seen the pet who sits too close to the fire. Some have eye complaints stemming from this, consider:

Aconite, Glonoinium, *Merc. sol.* and *Natrum sulph.*

EARS

Ears may conveniently be studied in two regions,

1 External ear and ear flap (see also skin).
2 Middle ear/Internal ear,

the most commonly occurring being trouble in the external ear canal. This is commonly but loosely referred to as canker. Since examination by auriscope is essential, treatment of the ear is best left to the veterinarian. Precipitating causes must be found and lesions in the ear canal identified to select a remedy.

All the usual procedures for examination and attention to problems e.g. excess hair, foreign body, etc. must be followed. Discharges and tissue debris can be removed by use of a proprietary natural debriding agent and parasites can be eliminated (see Ear Mites). Taking all such basic veterinary care for granted, homoeopathic treatment alone will be discussed here.

External Ear Canal

Ear Mites. Must be eliminated either by use of proprietary chemicals or preferably herbal insecticides or essential oils (they are not insects but are susceptible to similar substances). Red/brown wax, with or without pus, usually indicates the presence of ear mites. *Psorinum* or *Sulphur*, depending on the nature of discharges, are good homoeopathic remedies given internally to help remove the discharge and to render the environment hostile to mites. They may even serve to eliminate the infection by themselves. *Conium* is also useful, in this condition.

Foul Discharges, Pus etc. Many of the remedies affecting this condition are the deep acting polycrests which will work better if used at constitutional level of prescribing, but consider especially:

Arsen. alb., *Arsen. iod.*, *Calc. carb.*, *Calc. sulph.*, *Causticum*, *Graphites*, *Hepar sulph.*, *Kali bich.* (usually swollen ear canal and glands), *Kali carb.*, *Kali sulph.*, *Kreosotum*, *Mercurius* (canal inflamed, ulcers), *Psorinum*, *Pulsatilla*, *Rhus tox.* and *Sulphur*. If fishy discharges, *Sanicula* or *Tellurium*.

As usual, characteristic pointers to the remedies should be found, even if elsewhere in the body.

Disinfection of the ear by the use of essential oils can prove a very useful adjunct to treatment (see also Chapter 15).

Inflammation with Discharges

In early stages of inflammation	*Aconite*
If red, hot and swollen	*Belladonna*

Causticum, *Conium*, *Graphites*, *Kali bich.*, *Mercurius*, *Rhus tox.* and *Sulphur* are also very useful remedies.

If severe and sudden in the summer always suspect a grass seed. After removal use *Calendula* lotion or tincture in the canal to ease the pain and promote healing.

Ear Flap

Of less prescribing importance than discharge:

Haematoma	*Arnica, Hamamelis*
Scaly surface, scabby edge	*Tellurium*
Dry, scaly skin	*Arsen. alb.*, *Kali sulph.*
Dirty, smelly eczema around ear	*Psorinum*
Red, dry, itchy, worse warm room	*Sulphur*

Middle/Inner Ear

Usually manifested as a catarrhal deafness or loss of balance and holding head to one side. There can be eye movement (nystagmus) too. (**Age deafness** is a separate refractory problem but consider *Argent. met.*, *Causticum*, *Silica*, or *Thiosinaminum*). **The loss of balance** (see also p. 113) is helped by proper treatment of the external ear and by:

Staggering, trembling and weakness	*Gelsemium*
Falls when shakes head or tends to fall left	*Conium*
Better when lying down	*Cocculus*
When moving downwards	*Borax*
Tends to fall forwards	*Bryonia*
Falls to left	*Nat. mur.*
Falls to right	*Aconite*
	Causticum
Circles to the right	*Causticum*
Circles to the left	*Rhus tox.*

Catarrhal Deafness. Consider:

Agraphis nutans (especially cats), *Borax*, *Calcarea*, *Kali mur.* and *Pulsatilla*, according to particular and general symptoms.

Loss of balance (vertigo) as a result of middle or inner ear infection may be a good indication for the use of antibiotics to reduce the risk of damage. Homoeopathic remedies alone should not be relied upon to work fast enough here unless one is totally sure of one's ability. However, if you are experienced in the use of essential oils, these may dispense totally with the need for antibiotics when introduced into the ear canal. Acupuncture will help.

NOSE

Sneezing: **NB** Check for foreign body. If present or suspected give *Silica* unless it is easily retrievable. If not present:

With watery discharge	*Nat. mur.*, *Nux vom.*, *Sabadilla*

| With blood | Nitric acid |
| With itchy skin, worse with heat | Sulphur |

Snuffles:

Bland, creamy discharge, can be with blood	Pulsatilla
Corrosive discharge, nose blocked but runs	Arsen. alb.
Worse for warm room, worse at night	Nux vomica
Chronic	Calc. carb., Silica

Blocked Nose:

	Silica
Crusty blocked nose	Teucrum mar.
No discharge, but blocked up, voice altered	Sticta pulm.
With bleeding	Ipecacuanha
Worse for wet, cold weather	Rhus tox.
Yellow/Green thick discharge	Calc. fluor.
Yellow ropy catarrh	Kali bich.
With haemorrhage	Ferrum phos., Phosphorus

Cat 'flu: Is the specific nasal disease to consider in this section. Treat by nosode (if the patient is strong enough) with relevant similium and ensure that patient is not dehydrated through lack of water intake (see Chapter 11).

Debility afterwards, help build up with:

China, Ferrum phos. or *Phos. acid.*

Cracked Skin on nose:

| e.g. post Distemper | Nitric acid, Thuja |

Nose Bleeds (Epistaxis):

General remedy	Hamamelis
Sudden	Phosphorus
With sneeze	Carbo veg., Nitric acid
Especially if injury	Arnica
Blocked/Bleeding	Ipecacuanha
With vomiting	Eupatorium perfoliatum

| **Sores** ulcerated at edges of nostrils | Nitric acid |

Loss of Pigmentation (dogs especially).
No definitely indicated remedy. Try the trace elements:

Cobaltum, Cuprum, Ferrum, Iodum, Manganum and *Zincum.*

This is a condition of no known medical importance but does disfigure an animal from the show point of view. Seaweed or kelp supplements have also been tried with varying results. If the general health of the dog is restored and there is a good natural diet, pigmentation should return.

Sinuses: are functionally a part of the nasal system and all conditions of these are as for nasal symptoms.

MOUTH

Since the mouth is the opening of the alimentary canal and the respiratory system, it shares a common involvement with disease of the alimentary system and can show symptoms from the respiratory system. However it is entirely visible and therefore is a key area for picking up signs of disease.

Smell from the Mouth: This can originate from kidney disease, bad teeth, intestinal worms, ketosis, neoplastic conditions, throat disease, digestive disorder or mouth disease itself. As such, therefore, it is not useful in itself but only in the context of the whole animal.

Ulcerated Mouth: Where such ulcers are around the borders of mouth and skin, that is, on edge of lips consider *Nitric acid.*

Rodent Ulcer is to be found around the mouth and *Cistus can., Conium, Kali bich., Mercurius* and *Nitric acid* have all been found to be helpful (see also Skin). *Gallium aparine* Ø is of use topically and *Calendula* lotion. There also appears to be a hormonal link here as in miliary eczema and therefore one should consider:

Testosterone potentised, *Agnus castus* and *Ustilago maydis.* (See also pages 73 and 167.) Laser therapy may also prove useful (visible red wavelength).

Ulcers on tongue, palate, gums and inside cheeks. Consider:

Thirst, profuse saliva, sometimes vomiting and diarrhoea, puffy gums, sometimes with bleeding from gums, uraemic ulcers	*Mercurius sol.*
Blood from gums	*Phosphorus*
Kidney disease and uraemic ulcers	*Kali chlor.*
Slimy mouth	*Hydrastis*
Vesicles becoming usually well-circumscribed ulcers	*Borax*

Other remedies – *Arum triphyllum* and *Nitric acid*, and remember constitutional prescribing.

Profuse Salivation: When an animal shows profuse salivation it is a result of overproduction of saliva or of failure to swallow. Consider, in the latter case therefore, **Sore throats**: *Baryta carb.* (especially if the lymph glands are swollen in the neck), *Causticum, Hepar sulph., Lachesis, Merc. cyanatus, Merc. sol., Phytolacca* and *Silica* (see also p. 75).

Also consider:

Obstructed Throat – take appropriate action.

Tetanus (see also p. 130). Seek immediate veterinary attention.

Foreign Body in Mouth e.g. stick across the teeth – take appropriate action.

In the case of **Overproduction of Saliva** consider:

Baptisia, Lyssin, Mercurius, Pilocarpine and *Pulsatilla.*

Travel Sickness can present as drooling saliva (see p. 80).
Drooling may also be caused by disagreeable taste, fastidious appetite (especially cats) or reaction to a worming or antibiotic tablet. This is not pathological.

Underproduction of Saliva: Leads to a dry mouth. This is seen primarily in dehydration (rehydration therapy from your veterinary surgeon is essential) and in Key Gaskell Syndrome cats (see p. 134). Shock can also lead to a dry mouth, *Aconite* and *Arnica* may be helpful here. Where there is a dry mouth in association with other illness consider *Apis mel.*, *Arsen. alb.*, *Belladonna* or *Lycopodium.*

Sore Throats with dry mouths (as opposed to profuse salivation from sore throat on p. 74) lead one to think of:

Hot, painful, shiny throat, upset by noise, jarring or movement, red eyes	*Belladonna*
Constantly seeks fresh air, throat is grossly swollen and oedematous	*Apis mel.*
Dry mouth, with absence of thirst	*Pulsatilla*
Dry mouth with large thirst	*Arsen. alb.*

Gums can show ulceration (as for the mouth p. 73) and disease associated with the teeth – (see below). Remedies: *Apis, Arsenicum, Chamomilla, Kreosotum, Mercurius, Natrum mur., Nitric acid, Phosphorus.*

There is also the condition known as **Epulis** in which 'growths' are seen overlapping the teeth, consider here *Calc. carb.*, *Calc. fluor.* or *Thuja.*

Teeth

Tartar on the teeth leads to a foul mouth, receding gums, loose teeth, dental abscesses,* ulceration and pain. The teeth should be properly attended by a veterinarian, loose and diseased teeth being extracted and tartar removed. (It is usually possible to do this with a thumbnail in the conscious animal if not too advanced.) *Arnica* should be given before, during and after this operation. *Calendula* lotion should be used to soothe the sores and reduce the inflammation. *Fragaria* can be given to help prevent new tartar build-up, a few doses given every month will help. A raw bone should help to keep a dog's teeth clean but some dogs can create problems with bones. Cats can chew raw *organic* chicken wings or similar to maintain tooth and gum health. A

---

* Malar Abscess see p. 58.

mouthwash should be used to clean the teeth regularly. There are homoeopathic/herbal mouthwashes available. *Mercurial* remedies will aid recovery if there is much saliva and swollen gums.

In young dogs 'Teething' can be a problem. Here the remedy of choice is *Chamomilla* for all ills stemming from this teething state. Teething problems can affect any or all of the entire body system including the mental sphere. Apparently malicious chewing of furniture, etc. at this stage can be helped in some cases by *Chamomilla*.

Delayed Dentition, consider *Calc. carb.* or *Calc. phos.* Where there are defects in the enamel at this stage consider *Calc. fluor.* or *Fluoric acid.*

THE DIGESTIVE SYSTEM

The digestive system comprises the Oesophagus, Stomach, Intestines, Anus, Liver, Pancreas and the Mouth (already discussed). Vomiting, diarrhoea and constipation will also be included in this section.

Oesophagus

Dilated: This condition is seen in some young puppies and in Key Gaskell Syndrome (p. 134) in cats. Consider:

Alumina, Arsen. alb., Plumbum, Stramonium or *Veratrum album.* In many such cases, the remedies only help to maintain function, rather than cure.

Stomach

Hairball: Usually seen in cats only, it gives rise to digestive disturbances of a very general nature. Inappetance or increase of appetite, occasional vomiting, distended tummy and behavioural changes. It can be removed surgically but infinitely preferable is to help the cat either vomit it or pass it in the faeces if possible. Treatment according to symptoms can be very helpful, for example *Colocynth, Colchicum, Gratiola, Nux vomica* and *Raphanus.*

Ornithogallum Ø as a single dose can also be very helpful.

Foreign Bodies of any description in the stomach can be treated similarly.

Neoplastic disease of the stomach may be helped by using one of:

Arsen. alb., Asterias, Hydrastis, Ornithogallum Ø or *Phosphorus*.

Torsion of the Stomach. Surgery can be averted in some cases if one treats promptly with *Ornithogallum Ø* and *Colocynth* or *Colchicum* along with *Aconite*. If the dog is collapsed, give *Carbo. veg.* This condition is very serious and sudden and a **veterinarian should be consulted immediately**. There is usually no time to lose.

Hiccough: Especially in young puppies.

With eructation	*Nux vomica*
With yawning or nervous symptoms	*Ignatia*
With yawning	*Cocculus*

Pyloric Disorder: Passage of food on from the stomach is regulated by the pyloric sphincter. Stenosis of this organ, from injury, surgery or nervous causes, creates a functional obstruction, either partial or complete. *Staphisagria* is a remedy with particular effect on this structure, especially post-operatively. Consider also *Lycopodium, Nux vomica, Ornithogallum Ø* and *Phosphorus*. Acupuncture may help.

Intestines

Worms: Round worms – *Abrotanum, Cina, Chenopodium, Santoninum*.
Tape worms – *Filix mas., Granatum*.

It is not yet adequately proven that these remedies will cause the host to eliminate the parasite. If elimination of worms is required from a public health point of view, etc. unless proof can be found it would be unwise to rely totally on these remedies to do the job. Undoubtedly, however, the disease picture of parasitism can be greatly helped (possibly by restoring the host/parasite balance). Herbal preparations of these remedies are likely to be more effective in causing elimination (dosage levels need care) and *Garlic* also has a reputation in this field.

Work is urgently needed on this topic. Remember also *Alfalfa*, *Lecithin* or *Phos. acid* to aid build-up if debilitated.

Intussusception: Usually needs surgery, particularly if advanced, but 'symptomatic' homoeopathic treatment could help resolve the condition prior to surgery. Consider:

Chamomilla, Cina, Colchicum, Merc. cor., Nux vom. and *Veratrum album.*

Colic: This is abdominal pain. The accompanying symptoms help to guide one to the correct remedy.

Associated with teething in young animals	*Chamomilla*
With much tympany	*Colchicum,*
	Raphanus
After overeating	*Nux vomica*
Severe pain, back arched and abdomen cramped	*Colocynth*
Much reaction to noise and touch, with grinding	*Belladonna,*
of teeth	*Mag, phos.,*
	Zinc. met.
Flatus being passed	*Carbo veg.*
Grinding of teeth	*Cina, Plumb.*
	met., Podoph.
With stretching	*Dioscorea*

Foreign Body: Treat as for intussusception. This may aid the passage of the offending object and therefore may avert surgery. Do not delay consulting a veterinarian if symptoms are not relieved or if the condition appears serious. Beware maize (corn) cobs.

Flatulence: From either end of the digestive tract, consider:

If rich food is cause of trouble	*Nux vomica*
Due to vegetable material in diet	*Carbo veg.*

Also consider *Calc. carb., Lycopodium.*

Hernia: Herniation is the protrusion of abdominal contents (e.g. bowel) through a natural or accidental rupture in the body wall. The abdominal contents then lie beneath the skin. These hernias occur most commonly at the umbilicus, the inguinal region and the perineum. They are often caused by raised abdominal pressure and by an inherent weakness of the body wall.

Nux vomica or *Lycopodium* are indicated to try to help the underlying digestive causes and effects, they can even in some cases aid reduction of the hernia.

In cases of perineal hernia due to overstraining at the stool, consider *Alumina* or *Nux vomica*, but surgery may be necessary to restore proper function. Prostate (q.v.) treatment should be considered here too in male dogs.

A remedy closely associated with inguinal herniation is *Sulphuric acid*. Should the hernia become **incarcerated** or **strangulated** this is a very dangerous condition. Consider, as first aid, *Belladonna* and *Opium* and seek veterinary help urgently.

Veterinary advice should be sought with all forms of herniation.

Vomiting

This heading is not included under stomach conditions since the author believes that vomiting is such a potentially serious condition that it should be under a heading of its own. It is potentially serious for two reasons:

a) Loss of fluids and electrolytes leading to dehydration – a very dangerous condition possibly needing fluid therapy.
b) It may be a sign of some other severe illness such as Diabetes, Kidney trouble, Jaundice, Parvovirus and many others. It may also be the result of obstruction of the bowel.

Having said all this by way of caution, there can be many commonplace causes behind vomiting which, as long as the vomiting is not prolonged, need not be too serious. Carnivores will vomit naturally for their offspring. This, of course, requires no treatment.

By far the most common type of vomiting encountered is that of gastritis or gastroenteritis. Treat, as usual, in the homoeopathic manner, that is with regard to concomitant symptoms and the character of the vomit:

Mouth dry, often evidence of allergic reaction, seeks fresh air, absence of thirst.	*Apis mel.*
Simultaneous vomit and diarrhoea, (usually) dry mouth, very restless, may be blood in vomit or stool, clear white mucoid vomit (usually).	*Arsen. alb.*
Intolerance of milk in young animal. Milk often vomited as curds and animal can be shocked	*Aethusa*
Repeated reflex vomiting, such as seen in Parvovirus (see p. 129)	*Apomorphine*
Greenish bile vomited after large intake of water at one go. Thirst is for larger quantities at a time	*Eupatorium perfoliatum*
Large thirst, repeated cycles of drink/vomit, vomit usually yellow, mouth very wet with saliva	*Merc. sol.*
Large thirst, repeated cycle as above but usually more violent, vomit is usually watery/mucoid	*Merc. cor.*
Vomiting very soon after food	*Phosphorus*
Vomiting several hours after rich food (usually), stool may be absent or hard	*Nux vom.*
Vomiting several hours after fatty food (usually)	*Pulsatilla*
Simple regurgitation of food	*Ipecacuanha*
Frequent slimy vomiting with much retching and pain between bouts	*Ipecacuanha*
Immediate rejection of food with frothy yellow vomit at other times	*Veratrum alb.*
Post operative vomiting	*Nux vomica*

Where 'coffee ground' type vomitus is produced there is evidence of gastric bleeding and this is often of a serious nature, for example stomach neoplasia, ulcerated stomach. Think of *Ornithogallum* Ø for first aid. Consult a veterinary surgeon immediately.

Travel Sickness: May or may not be accompanied by vomiting but usually there is much drooling of saliva, a fearful or depressed expression of the face and an unwillingness to move.

Petroleum has proved to be very widely curative in this unfortunate and inconvenient condition. Think also of *Borax, Cocculus* and *Tabacum.* The misery of travel sickness to the dog and cat is difficult to imagine but should not be allowed to continue, as is often the case, simply because it is non serious and easily explicable. Do not smoke in the car as that can aggravate or cause the condition. Avoid fuel smells.

Diarrhoea

More common than vomiting and less often a symptom of serious illness but nonetheless the same words of caution should be applied when undertaking the treatment of diarrhoea (see p. 79). Again treat according to characteristics of the stool and concomitant symptoms.

In choosing a remedy one must consider several important questions. Is there straining before, during or after stool (tenesmus)? Is there flatus with stool? Is there abdominal pain? Is there pain on passing stool? Is the anus sore? Is the stool involuntary or without apparent sensation? One can detect this last symptom by the fact that the animal will pass stools without obvious discomfort and often in small quantities anywhere, anytime. A dog or cat is usually very particular about being clean in the house and, if 'caught short' by a sudden need to produce faeces, will usually produce near a door or on a particular floor surface or mat but *involuntary* stools are passed indiscriminately. For the purposes of this book, a distinction is not made between diarrhoea and dysentery.

Pasty diarrhoea, usually painless and non urgent	*Merc. sol.*
If there is tenesmus, with a forceful spurt of diarrhoea	*Merc. cor.*
Flatus and stool passed indiscriminately (spluttery) often so violently that the animal cannot control where it happens, often mucus with faeces. May also be involuntary leakage at anus	*Aloe*
Tenesmus, bloody or mucoid stools, often stools watery or frothy, often yellow, also	

tenesmus with no stool, often brought on by cold and wet conditions	*Rhus tox.*
Tenesmus, large quantities of stool and flatus produced at a time, stool may be yellowy and liquid or soft and loose	*Nat sulph.*
Diarrhoea with severe colic with arched back	*Colocynth*
Ineffectual urging and jelly like stools	*Colchicum*
Flatulent colic (frequently used in acute liver or pancreas conditions)	*Iris vers.*
Watery, greenish diarrhoea, especially in teething patient	*Chamomilla*
Watery, greenish diarrhoea	*Eupat. perf.*
When diarrhoea has semi-formed solid material in loose stool	*Calc. carb., Lycopodium, Ant. crud., Senecio*
When stool is loose, yellow and painless (usually), containing semiformed solid material	*Phos. acid*
When stool is black consider	*Crot. horr., Leptandra*
When there is much gurgling and stool is watery and forceful	*Croton tig., Podophyllum*
No two stools alike, patient shy, reserved and fussy feeder	*Pulsatilla*
Difficult to produce a small quantity of foul smelling faeces, which is partly formed with fluid, defaecation is painless (usually) but followed by great weakness. May be blood.	*Phosphorus*
Where great debility accompanies diarrhoea, usually with cold state with near collapse use	*Camphor, Veratrum alb., Carbo veg.*
When great debility accompanies diarrhoea also think of	*Bryonia Cuprum met., Rhus tox.*
Urgent stool giving rise to panic to produce stool	*Aloe, Causticum,*

	Croton tig.,
	Lilium tig.,
	Veratrum alb.
To help rebuild the constitution after	*China,*
debilitating diarrhoea	*Phos. acid*

Diarrhoea caused by various aetiological factors can be treated giving significance to those factors:

Severe fright	*Aconite*
General nervousness	*Argent. nit.,*
	Gelsemium
Injury	*Arnica*
Excessive intake of fruit	*Bryonia*
Excessive intake of rich food	*Nux vomica*
Teething	*Chamomilla*
Cold/wet	*Dulcamara,*
	Rhus tox.

Constipation: The failure of defaecation or difficulty in defaecation can be a useful guiding symptom in the choosing of a remedy or it can be a serious symptom in itself. Only while writing this section, I had cause to treat a Bassett Hound with quite severe post operative depression, painful urination, failure to pass faeces, vomiting with great distress (caused by overworking the abdominal wound during retching) and general malaise. *Nux vomica* was chosen, using the post operative constipation as a guiding symptom and within four hours the bitch had freely passed faeces (of a very hard nature) and had ceased vomiting. *Nux vomica* is also of help where there is much urging with the constipation, such as in the case of prostatitis with perineal herniation.

When stool cannot be passed with straining,	
whether the stool be soft or hard and dry	*Alumina*
When stool is large and painful and anus is red	
(often skin involvement and a dislike of heat)	*Sulphur*
'Shy' stool (i.e. stool which comes part way out	*Silica,*
and recedes)	*Thuja*

Very chalky stool, sometimes result of eating
bones   *Calc. carb.*
If liver dysfunction has given rise to constipation   *Sepia*
Post operative constipation   *Nux vomica*
Key Gaskell Syndrome   See p. 134

Anal Prolapse: Can occur with diarrhoea or constipation and depending upon concomitant symptoms, one should consider:

Aloe, Apis mel., Ignatia, Merc corr., Nux vomica, Podophyllum, Ruta grav. and *Sepia*.
If bleeding from the anus, *Aesculus* and *Nitric acid* are usually very effective.

Anal Furunculosis may be helped by *Calc. sulph., Hydrastis, Kali bich., Paeonia* or *Silica*.

Anal gland problems will be considered under skin troubles (see p. 106).

Liver and Pancreas

Problems of the liver and pancreas are usually of a severe enough nature to warrant **full veterinary attention**. Homoeopathic remedies can be extremely valuable.

For complaints of the **gall bladder** particularly think of *Berberis*.

General **liver** remedies are *Berberis, Chelidonium, Lycopodium* and *Nux vomica*. (See also Hepatitis q.v.)

Pain in the **liver** region, think of such remedies as *Aesculus, Chionanthus, Phosphorus* and *Sepia*.

Where there is **jaundice** think of:

Aesculus, Carduus mar., Chelidonium, Cuprum met., Hydrastis, Merc. sol. and *Phosphorus*.

Where the liver is overloaded by over-eating of **rich food**, *Nux vomica* is a great help.

The **pancreas** when diseased can give rise to two sets of problems, the first is digestive and the second metabolic.

a) **Pancreatic Insufficiency**: Gives rise to failure to digest fats and proteins in the bowel leading to diarrhoea which is usually yellow and pasty. Homoeopathic remedies can help here, consider *Chionanthus*, *Lycopodium* or *Senecio*. Diarrhoea and weight loss are associated with this condition and *Iodum* and *Phosphoric acid* fit these symptoms very well. It may still be necessary to supplement the diet with pancreatic enzymes for a while. Raw green tripe is also a good food, providing a supply of digestive enzymes as well as being a natural food for dogs.

b) **Diabetes Mellitus**: The failure of the insulin producing capacity of the pancreas gives rise to this condition which is a disturbance of the glucose metabolism in the tissue cells and the blood. Sugar also appears in the urine. *Insulin* in low potency along with *Iris versicolor*, *Phos. acid*, *Syzigium* or *Uranium nit.* can help to reduce symptoms and reduce urine sugar output. In some cases they can totally do away with the need for Insulin injections.

The pancreas can also suffer from acute inflammation (or **Pancreatitis**) and this is treated symptomatically. *Aconite*, *Atropinum*, *Iris versicolor* and *Phosphorus* can all help in this condition which is very painful, serious and troublesome.

THE URINARY SYSTEM

Conditions affecting any part of the urinary system, whose major function is the elimination of toxic materials and by-products from the blood, are potentially very dangerous and therefore **veterinary advice** should be sought in any such case. In this section only the homoeopathic treatment of such conditions shall be discussed, not the very important nursing and dietary aspects.

The most common conditions are inflammation of the kidney (Nephritis) and irritation of the bladder (Cystitis). The latter manifests itself as a frequent desire to urinate producing small quantities often, much tenesmus, pain and sometimes blood in the urine. This should not be confused with a blocked urinary system although the symptoms are similar. In the first there is usually an empty bladder and in the second a full bladder. Failure to distinguish correctly between the similar symptoms will lead to a tragic outcome so all pet owners should seek **veterinary advice**. Prostate problems in dogs may also present as urinary problems but must be distinguished (see Male Sexual System).

Cystitis

Burning pain, frequent attempts at micturition and bloody urine	*Cantharis*
Similar to above but less often indicated	*Merc. corr.*
Where overdistension is the cause of cystitis	*Causticum*
With neuromuscular involvement (e.g. post operative)	*Nux vomica* *Staphisagria*
Copious sediment in the urine	*Chimaphila*
Tenesmus and (sometimes) urinary incontinence, with much straining after urinating, can be haematuria	*Equisetum*

Blood in the urine, although usually symptomatic of urinary problems, may not always be so. Defects of the clotting mechanism or injury to the kidneys may also give rise to blood in urine. The latter one should treat with *Arnica*, the former (e.g. Warfarin poisoning) see Circulatory System.

As either the cause or effect of cystitis, **urinary calculi** can give rise to problems. They can create a blockage of the urinary system at any point but mostly this occurs in the male dog at the level of the os penis. It also occurs in bitches and dogs as a result of large stones blocking the neck of the bladder and in cats, especially male, in the urethra. *Calc. carb.*, *Calc. phos.* or *Lycopodium* should be a routine treatment of canine cases (while investigations are carried out) according to constitution. *Berberis*, *Benz. acid* or *Pareira* may also prove useful.

Sabulous plugs in the male cat respond well to *Sarsaparilla* and *Thlaspi bursa*.

When blockage has occurred as a result of injury and ensuing oedema, use *Arnica* and *Apis mel.*

Nephritis: This is a very difficult condition to treat in the advanced stages, but in the earlier stages responds well to such remedies as

Ammonium carb., *Arsen. alb.*, *Baptisia*, *Berberis*, *Kali chlor.*, *Mercurius*, *Nat. mur.*, *Plumbum met.*, *Phosphorus* and *Urtica urens*.

Since kidney problems are so serious, it is very necessary to know the various symptoms associated with these remedies to get a good result. This book has not the scope to cover these fully so you are referred to any good materia medica to obtain closer details. Some details are given in Chapter 17 to help match concomitant symptoms to remedies. **Veterinary attention** should always be sought.

Urinary Incontinence: This can occur as a result of cystitis (see p. 86) (cf. 'spraying' – see 'urination, inappropriate' p. 146), age or the ovarohysterectomy operation. With the latter I have had mixed success (possibly due to the animal no longer being 'normal') but try:

Calc. fluor., *Causticum*, *Nux vomica*, *Silica*, *Staphisagria* and *Thiosinaminum* from the physical point of view (see p. 96).
Stilboestrol in low potency, *Folliculinum*, *Sepia* or *Ustilago maydis* from the hormonal point of view.

For age incontinence try:

Agnus castus, *Causticum*, *Thiosinaminum* or *Turnera*.

I have found herbal treatments to be a useful support in cases of refractory incontinence.

MALE SEXUAL SYSTEM

The most frequent problem met in the surgery related to the male sexual system is a behavioural one: that of **Hypersexuality**. The young dog especially about 1½ to 2 years old becomes vagrant, peevish, over-boisterous, slightly unreliable and urinates territorially, including inside the house. This problem can also lead to prostate problems, cystitis, paraphimosis, injury from jumping fences and car accidents. The dog is generally antisocial and can suffer injury by the hand of offended owners of other dogs or property.

Remedies to consider are *Gelsemium*, *Lycopodium*, *Phosphorus*, *Tarentula hisp.* and *Zincum met.*

Weakness can occur as a result of this problem, consider *Conium* or *Picric acid*.

Although primarily female remedies, *Pulsatilla* and *Sepia* may help some dogs, according to constitution.

Where **convulsions** or extreme excitement with **salivation** occurs consider:

Chamomilla, Gelsemium, Ignatia, Lyssin, Nux vomica, Tarent. hisp. or *Zincum.*

Paraphimosis (prolonged erection with or without strangulation of the penis) can occur and here *Jacaranda, Picric acid* or *Selenium* can be of great help.

Prostatic problems are common and can occur in the older male dog for no apparent reason or the younger dog for the above reasons.

Older dogs may be helped by one of	*Agnus castus,*
	Conium,
	Ferr. pic.,
	Pulsatilla,
	Sabal serr.,
	Selenium
Where difficulty is encountered passing faeces	*Nux vomica,*
	Thuja
Where difficulty is encountered passing urine	*Merc. cor.,*
	Cantharis
With emissions of blood	*Ipecac, Nit. ac.*
Especially helpful to younger dogs	*Sabal serr.,*
	Staphysagria
Also helpful for younger dogs, especially with intermittent thin jets of urine often with skin complaints	*Clematis erecta*
Also helpful for the younger dog, especially if underweight and passes urine in a slow stream	*Baryta carb.*

Inflammation of the Penis and Prepuce occurs not infrequently and one should treat according to symptoms considering such remedies as:

Belladonna, Hepar sulph. and *Merc sol.*

(*Calendula* lotion infusions are often a great help and should not be forgotten for topical application on any sore inflamed area.)

Inflammation or Swelling of the Testicles is not often seen but depending on the cause and appearance one can treat with:

In case of injury	*Arnica,*
	Bellis perennis
When acute inflammation is present	*Aconite,*
	Belladonna,
	Pulsatilla,
	Rhododendron
When the testes are indurated and smaller than normal (usually in the aged dog) consider	*Agnus castus,*
	Clematis,
	Conium,
	Iodum

Retained Testicle, Monorchidism or Cryptorchidism are seen fairly frequently.

One should think in terms of:

Baryta carb., Calc. carb., Clematis, Testosterone in low potency and *Thyroidinum.*

One should take care to minimise influence from oestrogenic chemicals.

Deficient Sexual Power is mostly noticed in the stud dog and is rare.

Testosterone in low potency can help as can *Agnus castus, Conium, Lycopodium, Phos. acid, Sabal serr.* and *Selenium.*

Where the penis is extruded but desire is absent try *Yohimbinum.*

Infertility. Take especial note of nutrition and diet. Consider constitutional prescribing in support.

The Castrated Male Dog and Cat have their own particular problems.

DOG   Bilateral hair loss on the sides of the body and problems with overweight predominate. One should always consider *Testosterone* in low potency and *Agnus castus*. Food intake should be restricted if obesity is occurring (see Obesity p. 126 and Female p. 96).

Where problems of **hair loss** are encountered one should consider, apart from *Testosterone*:

Thallium acetas, *Thyroid* in low potency and *Ustilago maydis*.

CAT Skin problems are of especial importance here, the most common being 'Miliary Eczema'. *Progesterone* or *Testosterone* in low potency should be considered as too should *Pulex*, the potentised flea, which can help in some cases. The lesions' character should also help to guide one to homoeopathic remedies here. For example:

Antimonium crud., *Antimonium tart.*, *Arsen. alb.*, *Cicuta*, *Dulcamara*, *Graphites*, *Lycopodium*, *Mezereum*, *Muriatic acid*, *Natrum mur.*, *Phosphorus*, *Rhus tox.*, *Sepia*, *Sulphur*, *Thallium* and *Zinc. met.* have all been used with varying success. **Think constitutionally** (see also p. 157 and p. 159).

As a general rule many problems associated with neutering in the cat or dog, male or female, seem to be difficult to treat homoeopathically and a few appear to be completely refractory. One could hypothesise that the patient is no longer normal and homoeopathy works best through the normal system. However, with persistence, success often ensues.

FEMALE SEXUAL SYSTEM

Under this umbrella are gathered conditions affecting the ovaries, womb and mammary glands, fertility problems, problems of pregnancy, parturition and motherhood and finally lactation. The part the female plays in the continuation of life in mammals is far greater than that played by the male, so this heading will embrace many more topics and much more information than was contained in the section on the male. More problems are encountered in bitches than in queens.

Ovaries, Cyclicity, Infertility, Behavioural Problems associated with Ovarian Cycle:
Remedies (note that these are constitutional prescriptions since that is the best approach in my experience) having a particular effect on the

functioning of the ovaries, on the behaviour associated with this and on fertility are:

Sepia
A remedy for the bitch who is moody, morose, over protective, sometimes vicious. This description fits the symptoms of false pregnancy in many bitches and should always be considered in this condition. The bitch can be unwilling to mate. Improves in open air.

Pulsatilla
Is a remedy to be used in similar connections to *Sepia* but much more open, sunny natured, yielding type of bitches who are up and down in their moods, show a variable appetite and have a shy nature. Variability is the byword of Pulsatilla (the wind flower) and variable it is in this context. A creamy vulval discharge is often present after oestrus.

Platina
For the haughty detached mentality, who can be highly strung.

Lachesis
Is very much like *Sepia*. It has a predilection for the throat area, and for the left side of the patient. Jealousy is predominant in the symptoms, and suspicion. There is often much bleeding of dark blood at oestrus and the mammary glands can show a purplish tinge.

Iodum
Can be of use, particularly in thinner subjects, to encourage a bitch to display oestrus, if retarded.

Natrum mur.
A timid and withdrawn type which seeks solace in her own company when unwell. The bitch or queen has a liking for salt and dislikes strong sunlight. At mating, behaviour can be unwilling and aggressive.

Palladium
Is effective in those who brighten-up enormously when with the carer for going out but sink into apathy when left alone. It is a right sided remedy.

Lilium tig.
Suits the overanxious, depressed bitch who is always on the move. Often there is a rheumatic appearance to the walk. This animal does not enjoy a fuss and likes to be left alone.

Murex
Applies mostly to queens and rarely to bitches when a condition of nymphomania is present, that is, she is

repeatedly calling. She is always lively, nervous and affectionate. *Ferula glauca*, *Gratiola* and *Origanum* should also be remembered in this connection.

I shall refer to many of these predominantly female constitutional remedies again and again in this section so refer back to these pages for clarification of the indications for use of the remedies (also Chapter 17).

After the heat period in the bitch a '**false pregnancy**' period is usual. This may or may not show itself but can display anything from nearly no signs to a full imitation of the pregnant state from conception to birth, including mammary development with milk during the supposed nursing period. More often than not, when there are signs, they are of a moody disposition with variable milk production. Often a 'nest' is made and the bitch guards it. *Sepia* or *Pulsatilla* according to the disposition of the bitch could be used. To aid the drying up of secretions of milk, do not massage the glands but give remedies such as *Bryonia*, *Calc. carb.*, *Cyclamen*, *Pulsatilla*, *Sepia* and *Urtica* (the latter in low potency).

Also after the heat period, often about six weeks later, a bitch may become polydypsic and off colour. There may or may not be a vaginal discharge. This heralds the condition **pyometra** which is potentially exceedingly serious and can require ovarohysterectomy. In severe stages the bitch can become toxic, dehydrated, suffer kidney damage and even die.

Homoeopathic treatments in the earlier stages can help tremendously but veterinary advice should be sought. Remedies such as *Aletris*, *Caulophyllum*, *Pulsatilla*, *Sabina* and *Sepia* and, in cases where there is toxicity and vomiting, *Echinacea*, have all been used with degrees of success varying in effect from 100 per cent to insufficient to avert surgery. Much must depend on the speed of onset, the severity and the duration before treatment. *Pulsatilla* is not so likely to be used for this condition since *Pulsatilla* patients rarely display great thirst.

Problems of Pregnancy, Parturition and the Post Partum Period. More of this text applies to the bitch than the queen although remedies are as effective in either. It appears however that the bitch needs more attention than the queen at this time. It is worth remembering that when any creature is pregnant, be that creature human, canine, feline or whatever, any food, drug, vaccine, etc. administered will affect both mother and offspring. It is here that homoeopathy has especial advantage over conventional medicine (see also Preventive Medicine in Chapter 14). One should always avoid vaccinations during this sensitive period and try to avoid the use of any drugs.

Pregnancy in the bitch and queen is usually uneventful but *Caulophyllum* should always be given towards the end of pregnancy (about three times weekly for the last two weeks) to ease the impending birth process. Where abortion is threatened *Viburnum* has a great reputation and one can also use the *nosodes* of any specific infective agents, which may be involved in the cause, to prevent abortion. *Cobaltum nitricum* also has a reputation where repeated abortion occurs in an individual. Debility after abortion can be helped by *Kali carb.*

During the birth process *Caulophyllum* is again indicated and *Calc. phos.* to improve the tonicity of the womb. Any difficulties at this stage can be dramatically helped by these remedies. *Pulsatilla* and *Sepia* can also be used to help some of the mental side of the problem. *Gossypium* or *Secale* can be of value when a bitch giving birth to a lot of puppies becomes exhausted (also think of *Cuprum acet.* in these circumstances).

Should a Caesarean section be necessary despite these efforts, remember *Arnica*, *Secale* and *Staphisagria* to aid the post-operative recovery (see also Post Operative Remedies p. 126).

When a delivery has been traumatic for the mother, always remember *Bellis per.*; or possibly *Apis mell.* where urination is difficult as a result of oedema. Remember the offspring too. *Arnica* is of great value here and consider *Baryta carb.*, *Helleborus*, *Hypericum*, *Laurocerasus* and *Nat. sulph.* where necessary (see materia medica, Chapter 17 and Injury p. 123). Sometimes offspring and mother suffer from the anaesthetic administered and one should bear in mind the relevant potentised anaesthetic and *Opium*. When a puppy or kitten is cold and collapsed use *Carbo veg.* (see also Puppy Problems p. 147).

Post partum involution of the womb and expulsion of membranes and debris is encouraged by *Caulophyllum*.

Haemorrhage post partum is rarely a problem in the dog and cat but can be helped by the following remedies according to the character of the bleeding (see Haemorrhage p. 121 and Materia Medica):

Aconite	*Hamamelis*	*Phosphorus*
Aletris	*Ipecacuanha*	*Sabina*
Crocus	*Lachesis*	*Secale*
Crotalus	*Millefolium*	*Thlaspi bursa*
Ferrum met	*Nitric acid*	*Ustilago*

Retained Afterbirth is also rare but consider:

Caulophyllum, Lilium tig., Pulsatilla, Sabina, Sepia or *Ustilago*. Think constitutionally.

If toxaemia arises, consider *Echinacea* or *Pyrogen*.

Mismothering or a failure of the maternal behaviour to correctly 'switch on' consider:

Lachesis, Lilium tig., Platina, Pulsatilla or *Sepia*.

They have all been used successfully, using the homoeopathic method for selection of a remedy (see p. 90).

Failure to produce enough milk for the puppies or kittens is a relatively more common condition. Consider here such remedies as:

Calc. carb., Calc. phos., Lecithin, Medusa and *Urtica* (the latter in high potency).

Conium, Iodum and *Sabal serr.* will encourage an underdeveloped mammary gland.

A few days after giving birth several conditions may arise:

Eclampsia, a disturbance of the Calcium metabolism occurs in some cases and is characterised by a range of symptoms from restlessness through to collapse in tetany. There is usually very rapid breathing. *Calc. phos.* and *Mag. phos.* are primary remedies here. *Arsen alb., Belladonna, Cicuta, Hyoscyamus, Ignatia, Lilium tig., Stramonium* and *Zinc.* can all be used according to symptoms and *Hydrocyanic acid* where there is much cyanosis. Intravenous injection of Calcium is a must, if symptoms are severe or prolonged, since the mother can die from this condition. **Veterinary attention** is essential. *Calc. phos.* given prior to confinement can help avoid this condition.

Mastitis can develop soon after parturition or after weaning. Here think of:

Apis mell, Belladonna, Bryonia, Lachesis, Phytolacca or *Urtica,* according to symptoms shown. There are several proprietary compounds on sale in France and Germany where various of these are mixed together. This precaution is to avoid the risk of failure due to incorrect prescribing and a high success rate is claimed (but see p. 44). **Veterinary attention** should be sought (see also p. 44).

Metritis is an inflammation, and probably an infection, of the womb following parturition and usually shows a vulval discharge. According to the condition of the mother and the character or odour of the discharge, one should consider:

Caulophyllum, Pulsatilla, Sabina, Secale, Sepia and *Ustilago.*

Remember also:

Baptisia, Echinacea or *Pyrogen* if septicaemia or toxaemia results.

Nipples can exhibit some problems, for example cracked and sore nipples from sucking puppies or kittens consider *Graphites* by mouth and *Calendula* lotion on the nipples.

Inverted Nipples can he helped by *Sarsaparilla* or *Silica* and these remedies should be given in limited doses before the end of pregnancy or, better, before mating if the condition is noticed at the time.

Weaning puppies or kittens can result in the mother having too much milk and the mammae becoming engorged. The flow of milk can be reduced with low potency *Urtica* or *Cyclamen* but be warned of mastitis developing as a result of this engorgement of the glands. Consider also *Conium. Ignatia* will help the mental problems associated with weaning (for problems in offspring at this time see p. 148) and

Calc. carb., *China*, *Kali carb.* or *Lecithin* will help to build up body condition again.

Mammary Tumours (see also p. 125) may develop in older bitches and queens, whether or not they have had puppies or kittens. Homoeopathy makes no extravagant claims that it can cure these completely, but they can in some cases be controlled and, in a few cases cured. The following remedies all have a reputation in this field:

Arsen. alb., *Asterias*, *Calc. fluor.*, *Calc. iod.*, *Chimaphila*, *Conium*, *Hydrastis*, *Phosphorus*, *Phytolacca*, *Schirrinhum*, *Scrophularia* and *Thuja*.

One should think of *Phosphorus* where there is suppuration and *Asterias* if there is ulceration. Remember constitution and diet. Benign growths paradoxically may be more difficult to treat than malignancies.

Problems of the Ovarohysterectomy Female. They are MILIARY ECZEMA in cats (see p. 90 but think of low potency *Oestrogen* and *Progesterone*) and in bitches OVERWEIGHT and URINARY INCONTINENCE. OBESITY leads one to think of *Calc. carb.* or *Pulsatilla* as a remedy but where there is a tendency to skin trouble as well think of *Graphites* or *Sulphur*. *Ant. crud.* or *Anacardium* can help real gluttons. ALOPECIA (q.v.) may also be a problem.

URINARY INCONTINENCE as a result of 'spaying' can be a very refractory condition to treat. Consider *Oestrogen* in low potency or *Causticum*, *Gelsemium*, *Sabal serr.*, *Turnera* or *Ustilago* (see also p. 87).

RESPIRATORY SYSTEM

Upper Respiratory Problems commonly encountered are coughs, cat flu (see nose), sinusitis (see nose), sore throats (see mouth) and laryngitis (which usually takes the form of a changed 'voice').

Lower Respiratory Problems include difficulty in breathing and coughs.

Cough. This is usually the response to irritation in the larynx, trachea or lungs as a result of foreign body aspiration or inflammation from, for example, infection. Beware however of the 'heart' type of cough (see heart) or worms. Upper respiratory coughs are generally less serious than lower respiratory coughs and generally a harsher sound but always, in homoeopathy, one treats according to the symptoms not the diagnosis of specific diseases. Beware of the potentially serious nature of some coughs. **Veterinary advice** should be sought if at all in doubt.

Dogs and cats rarely display the character of sputum so all there is to go on usually is the type of cough and the modalities. Major remedies are:

Dry spasmodic cough	*Belladonna, Bryonia, Cuprum, Drosera, Pertussin, Stannum, Sticta*
Cough with vomit	*Ipecacuanha*
Cough with retching	*Drosera, Nux vomica*
Hoarseness	*Bryonia* (worse for movement), *Causticum, Phosphorus*
Dry teasing cough	*Aconite, Nux vomica, Pulsatilla, Rhus tox.*
Rattling cough	*Ant. tart., Dulcamara, Ferrum phos., Stannum*
Choked cough	*Spongia*
With dyspnoea	*Ammon. carb., Ant. tart., Arsen. alb., Kali carb., Lycopodium, Phosphorus, Spongia*
With fluid mucus	*Coccus*

If **Kennel Cough** (Canine tracheobronchitis) is suspected then in addition to the similium remember the *nosode* (see Chapter 11).

Asthmatic breathing	*Apis mell.* (a strong desire for fresh air, usually lung congestion. *Arsen. alb.* (restless). *Aspidosperma Ø, Lobelia inflata, Spongia* (worse for heat), *Sulphur* (worse for heat and usually skin problems too)

Asphyxia   *Ant. tart.* (phlegmy and blue),
              Apis mell. (if oedema of throat is cause),
              Carbo veg. (blueness and very cold with
              collapse), *Laurocerasus* Ø (blueness).
              Always use *Aconite* intercurrently.

All these symptoms of cough and troubled breathing may be a result of heart problems and are, therefore, potentially very serious. Consult your **veterinary surgeon.**

Cat 'flu see Chapter 8 – Nose, and Chapter 11 – Specifics.

N.B. Smoking in the house can lead to serious aggravation of or even cause respiratory problems for your animal companion.

THE HEART, CIRCULATORY SYSTEM AND BLOOD

In all cases of heart trouble **veterinary advice** should be sought as the professional can best assess cardiac problems and their response to treatment. The following remedies have been found to be of use.

In case of heart weakness	*Crataegus* Ø,
	Digitalis in low potency,
	Strophanthus Ø.
In cases of heart cough	*Naja,*
	Prunus v.,
	Spongia
In cases of Angina	*Aconite* with:
	Cactus or
	Cimicifuga
Thudding heart	*Lycopus*
In cases of Arrhythmia	*Convallaria* Ø
If heart is slow and pulse weak, valvular conditions, heart often oversized	*Viscum album*
Valvular disorders with ascites	*Adonis vernalis*
In cases of cyanosis	*Laurocerasus* Ø

In cases of **acute failure** there is much distress. Here *Aconite, Ant. tart., Arsen. alb.* and *Carbo veg.* can help the situation according to the symptoms.

Ascites or Dropsy is the name given to the accumulation of fluid in the abdomen. This can arise from several causes (see Feline Infectious Peritonitis pp. 132–133 and Lymphatic System below) but is commonly caused by right ventricular heart failure or by a swollen liver.

Adonis vernalis, *Apis mell.*, *Apocynum* and *Digitalis* have all been used with degrees of success. All these remedies have a strongly diuretic action and, with the exception of *Apis*, help the heart directly too. Herbal diuresis may be valuable to assist treatment.

Pulmonary Congestion from a similar problem on the left side of the heart is greatly helped by *Apis mell.*, *Arsen. alb.* and *Spongia* (see also Asthmatic Breathing p. 97). Herbal diuresis may be valuable to assist treatment.

Anaemia and Haemorrhage see Generalities pp. 119 and 121.

THE LYMPHATIC SYSTEM
(RETICULO-ENDOTHELIAL SYSTEM)

This consists of the lymph ducts alongside all the veins, the lymph nodes at various sites in the body and the major lymphatic duct back to the heart. Their function is to drain from the tissues fluid which has left the blood vessels. They also form an important part of the defence mechanisms of the body, supplying antibody defences and defensive filtration in the lymph nodes. The spleen, bone marrow and liver are also involved and the thymus in the very young. The tonsils are also an important part of this system (see Sore Throats p. 75).

Generalised swelling of all the lymph glands can be helped by:

Arsen. alb., *Arsen. iod.*, *Arum triph.*, *Baryta iod.*, *Calc. fluor.*, *Cistus can.*, *Iodum* and *Lapis albus* according to symptoms.

If it is a form of lymphosarcoma that is manifesting itself in this way, then the prognosis may be grave. However, many such cases have responded to careful homoeopathic management.

Lymph nodes swollen in the throat region often accompanied by a sore throat (see p. 75) may be helped by *Mercurius*, *Baryta* and *Calc. fluor.* For indurated glands think of *Cistus*, *Conium* or *Lapis*.

When lymph nodes in particular parts of the body (e.g. inguinal region) are enlarged it is usually a sign of neoplasia or infection in the parts distal to that gland. **Veterinary inspection** is helpful.

For infected parts use *Hepar sulph.* Neoplasia presents greater problems (see p. 124).

LOCOMOTOR SYSTEM

(Which is taken to mean all parts of the musculo-skeletal system apart from the head, which has already been mentioned p. 57).

Skeletal Problems – Bones and Joints

Young dogs (and, more rarely, cats) can suffer from incorrect bone metabolism leading to large epiphyseal swellings ('knobbly' legs and ribs), bone deformities as a result of softening and often lameness. The joints fail to form correctly and permanent disability throughout life can result. Calcium and other mineral supplementation and vitamins A, C and D are known to help control the problem and overall diet is important. Homoeopathically one can help tremendously with *Calc. phos.* or *Calc. fluor.* (see also p. 148).

Calc. carb. is more useful if the puppy is very fat or flabby in appearance.

Silica also helps to form connective tissues properly and can be a long term help. In the very debilitated puppy or kitten use *Phos. acid* as well.

Phos. acid should always be remembered in debility, especially in rapidly growing, undernourished, overstrained young patients.

Where sore joints are suspected remember *Ruta grav.* and excessive exercise should be avoided.

In older pups nearing adulthood, where one can see that they are late developers use:

In lean dogs	*Calc. phos.*
In those still with puppy fat and physically soft, to help complete their maturity	*Calc. carb.*

In the mentally backward	*Baryta carb.*
Where they have clearly outgrown themselves (i.e. incoordination between growth and development) and are threatened by over exertion (there is a great temptation to over exercise the young undermature dog)	*Calc. fluor., Phos. acid*

Dwarfism, a separate problem, may be helped by *Baryta carb.*, *Iodum*, *Thuja* or *A.C.T.H.* in potency.

Bony Lumps (exostoses) are not uncommon (often as a result of previous trauma) and the treatment of choice here is usually *Hekla lava*, but consider also *Calc. fluor.* and *Silica* (see also Head p. 57).

Another 'nutritional' syndrome is that occurring in kidney disease, often called **osteodystrophy**, which manifests itself as a softening of the bone. It results from impaired mineral metabolism as a result of malfunctioning kidneys. Treat the patient constitutionally (and see Kidneys p. 87).

An excellent remedy for toughening the bone and helping mineralisation is *Calc. fluor. Hekla lava* also helps in this respect.

Osteoporosis is a demineralisation of bone occurring with age. Similar treatment is advisable remembering also *Calc. carb.*, *Calc. phos.* and *Silica*. Correct nutrition is vitally important.

Osteomyelitis is an inflammation, usually from infection, of the medulla of the bone. **Veterinary attention** should be sought.

Hepar sulph. and *Kali iod.* are of paramount importance here in controlling infection and then consider helping the bone tissues with *Ruta grav.* (periosteum), *Calc. fluor.* (bone itself) and *Symphytum*. The relevant *nosode* is also very helpful.

Fractures of Bone (see also Injury p. 123) are always helped by *Symphytum* and *Ruta grav.* Use of these remedies will usually prevent the 'non-union; phenomenon. *Calc. phos.* and *Silica* also help the bone metabolism. One should always remember the mental and soft tissue effects of broken bones and give *Aconite* if there is a lot of fear and always *Arnica*.

Injury to Bone which doesn't cause a fracture can lead to exostoses (see p. 101) but *Arnica* and *Ruta* will help to prevent any such occurrence. *Symphytum* is also of value (see also Injury p. 123). If exostoses occur, use *Hekla*.

Injury to Joints (see also Injury p. 123) always remember *Arnica* with *Rhus tox.* and *Ruta grav.*

Luxation (dislocation) of joints is a serious injury but after reduction treat as above.

Subluxation is the name given to poorly formed joints which do not articulate correctly. A classical example here is **Hip Dysplasia**. In this condition the ball and socket joint of the hip varies from slightly abnormal (on X-ray) to extremely shallow and almost non-existent. This is another case of growth/development incoordination. The result is hind leg weakness and arthritis. *Colocynth* and the appropriate 'arthritic' treatment (see below) help enormously. Remember too *Calc. carb.* or *Calc. phos.* in young dogs. Some small breeds have a similar problem with the **Patella** (knee cap) and I have found *Gelsemium* to help this condition, again with the appropriate 'arthritis' remedy should secondary arthritis be present. (Subluxation may also occur as a result of injury.)

Spinal Problems (see also Hind Leg weakness (p. 104) and Paralysis p. 106).

Disc lesions, lumbar spasm and any other pain in this region	*Berberis v.,* *Nux vomica*
Where urination is difficult	*Causticum*
Where defaecation is difficult, with muscular spasm	*Nux vomica*

Also *Hypericum, Plumbum, Phosphorus* and *Ruta grav.* have been found to be helpful. This condition occurs especially in Dachshunds. *Angustura vera* is also a useful adjunct to treatment to prevent nerve damage. Such patients should be resolutely rested and, after the acute stage, help may be sought from an Osteopath or Chiropractor.

Acupuncture also has a great reputation in this field, and can prove invaluable. The author has enjoyed good success with acupuncture and homoeopathy combined.

Where arthritis of the vertebrae or exostoses are considered to be instrumental in the cause of the condition think also of *Causticum, Hekla lava, Rhus tox.* and *Ruta grav.*

Inflammation of the joints, known by the emotive name of **Arthritis**, produces varying symptoms both locally in the joints and generally (manifested in lameness). Much is lost to the veterinary homoeopath in this sphere in that 'character of pain' is an important prescribing point in human homoeopathy, but that cannot be divined in animals. Local signs at the joint include swelling, pain on palpation, deformation, pain on movement of joint, fluid, skin changes, etc. The lameness varies in its symptoms and this variation is especially important. Many questions need to be asked, for example: Is the lameness worse for movement or better for movement, worse with heat or cold or better for heat or cold? Is it worse at the end of a rest after long period of exercise? Does the lameness seem to bother the animal badly or is it just a nuisance? Is it the result of a specific injury? Has the patient a temperature indicating infected arthritis (here the relevant *nosode* would be a useful adjunct to any symptomatic treatment e.g. Streptococci, Staphylococci)? Is it an acute arthritis or a chronic longstanding case? (see also Post Op. p. 126).

Acute and chronic arthritis are not treated as separate entities but one would use different dosage regimes. One would not expect a very rapid cure in a chronic case and would use less frequent dosing, but one would require rapid response in an acute case (thereby preventing the tendency to become chronic) so would give frequent doses in a day. Both cases would be treated according to symptoms. In **infected** cases remember the *nosodes* with *Hepar sulph.* along with *Aconite* or *Belladonna* in acute cases and *Silica* in chronic cases. *Ledum* is indicated if an injury with a sharp penetrating object has occurred, and *Arnica* in any case of injury. *Rhus tox.* and *Ruta grav.* are also very good remedies in injury to joints, aiding healing of the fibrous tissues and prevention of adverse sequelae. Diet is of especial importance in the management of arthritis.

'Symptomatic'* Treatment of Arthritic Problems: (see also Muscular Problems p. 105 and Chapter 17).

Rhus tox.	Joint pain and lameness worse just after rest and especially after resting and after exercise. The patient 'limbers up' and lameness can disappear entirely on exercise. This does not mean a patient must be vigorously exercised since, in the long run, failure to rest or be steady will lessen the chances of healing. Patients are also worse in cold damp weather.
Bryonia	This is the second remedy of great repute in this condition. Its symptoms are worse for movement and warmth. At first sight it is the exact opposite of *Rhus tox.* and it is for this reason that these two remedies above all others are commonly assumed to cover the whole spectrum of arthritis symptoms. This is however, far from the case. Where neither is indicated many others can fit the picture.
Dulcamara	Symptoms worse in changeable Autumn weather (and to a lesser extent, Spring), worse at night, similar to *Rhus* in response to movement. Skin and diarrhoea symptoms may coexist.
Caulophyllum	Usually in the small joints and can often start up in pregnancy. The neck can also be affected, often worse turning to the left.
Calc. phos.	Suits those growing pains that can so often trouble the 6 to 12 month old dog. Also conditions of the joints which arise in pregnancy (see also *Caulophyllum*).
Causticum	Severe pain, sometimes joint deformities, weakness of muscles tending almost to paralysis. Unsteadiness of legs. Better with damp warmth, worse dry cold.
Colchicum	Worse for movement and in warm weather (see also *Bryonia*) and at night. Oedema of legs.

* This term is used in this text to imply selection of a homoeopathic medicine according to the symptoms displayed. This is only an aide-memoire and should not override 'constitutional' considerations to which the symptoms can be a pointer.

Where visible changes occur at the joints consider:

Apis	Oedematous swelling of joints, skin has a shiny appearance worse for heat, touch and pressure and desires fresh air. Better for cold bathing.
Colchicum	Swellings of joints and joint deformities.
Calc. fluor., *Hekla lava.*	Where exostoses are evident.

No specific mention has been made of such conditions as **Osteochondritis Dissecans** since 'symptomatic' remedies (as above) and rest, within one's capabilities, are usually sufficient treatment. OCD is a further manifestation of growth/development incoordination with over-exuberant exercise taking a toll of the vulnerable tissues. Refer to p. 100 for help to correct that weakness.

Muscular Problems

Injury (trauma) to muscles should always receive *Arnica* or *Bellis perennis* (especially the pelvic area). One should also remember, in the case of tendons, *Rhus tox.* and *Ruta grav.*

Overexertion (and therefore fatigue and bruising) indicates *Arnica*. Pulled muscles also require *Rhus tox.*

In the case of the overworked dog remember too *Calc. phos.* or *Phos. acid*. The trauma of parturition can be treated with *Bellis* in preference to *Arnica*, or with *Apis mell.* if perineal oedema.

'Rheumatic' conditions should be treated in a similar way to arthritic conditions (i.e. according to symptoms) and many of the remedies are used for either (often a differential diagnosis is academic) see p. 104. However, where no apparent joint involvement can be detected, serious disability can occur and a few **extra** remedies can be called into play:

Pains worse for cold, better for warmth especially stiffness of neck and back. There is usually marked agitation with varying degrees of weakness	*Cimifuga rac.* (*Actaea rac.*)

A classic old dog remedy, indicated by a progressive weakness of the hind legs for no apparent reason	*Conium*
Shows similar signs to *Conium*, but the joints are often affected	*Lithium carb.*
Showing progressive weakness of the limbs, joints can be affected. Shakes.	*Causticum*
Similar but often with alopecia	*Thallium*

Tendency to paralysis (see also CDRM (p. 114))

Where one group of muscles in particular is involved	*Plumbum*
Where a widespread paralysis is evident, usually of a spastic nature (see also Fits p. 112)	*Lathyrus*
Where 'rheumatism' has led to paralysis	*Causticum, Rhus tox., Phosphorus*
Where spinal problems are suspected	*Conium, Lathyrus*
Where spinal problems are suspected in hypersexual states.	*Picric acid*

Muscular trembling (cross reference here with Nervous System)

Old dogs	*Calc. phos., Causticum, Kali phos., Phosphorus*
Excitement	*Mercurius*
Anticipation	*Kali brom.*
Exertion	*Rhus tox.*
After defaecation, usually in older dogs	*Conium*

SKIN

In the realm of skin disease it is true to say that homoeopathic treatment does not produce a rapid cure nor cure every case. However, the successes are very encouraging, despite the time often taken. Efforts to take the work of this section further can only improve the situation. Two reasons leap to mind to explain the difficulties. One is the likelihood that, since animal skin is so different from human, remedies would have different provings in animals with regard to skin symptoms. The other is the very important fact that the skin is the largest organ of the body, and although only able to manifest disease in a few ways, more often than not reflects a deep internal problem, the nature of which is not easy to detect, especially in animals. This is usually ultimately an immune imbalance but it manifests itself in mental and physical signs. The all too obvious skin problems are seen, but it is very difficult to look beyond to see the whole patient internal problem from which they arise, even if it is suspected that such a problem exists, for modern medicine tends to think mostly in terms of contact allergy, ectoparasites, bacterial or fungal infections, dermatitis from chemical irritants, hormonal problems, trauma and self inflicted trauma (see Appendix 8). It is when one opens one's mind to the vast 'dustbin' of 'idiopathic' skin diseases (those arising from no apparent cause) that one starts to search around for involvement within the animal's immune function, metabolism and psyche. The skin is a whole body organ and is very sensitive to whole body conditions. Thus, sometimes, the **only** symptoms of disease of the whole body are skin symptoms. The answer to more effective homoeopathic skin treatment and more consistent success must lie in remembering this and in striving to seek the correct *constitutional* remedy to correct the underlying imbalance.

When psychological (mental) causes for skin complaints (whatever the symptom) are suspected refer to Chapter 12 on Mental Conditions.

When after-effects (sometimes long lived) or specific infectious diseases are suspected use the relevant *nosode*.

When after-effects of vaccination are suspected, again use the relevant *nosode* and consider *Pulsatilla*, *Sulphur* or *Thuja* very strongly when seeking a constitutional remedy (see p. 159). Vaccination may be a common trigger for skin problems, most of which can be observed to have started within three months after a vaccination event. *Ledum* and *Silica* should also be considered.

When hormonal problems are suspected, use the relevant hormone in potency and *Iodum*, *Ustilago* or *Thallium* along with the relevant 'symptomatic'* and constitutional remedies.

Where metabolic problems are suspected (e.g. in liver dysfunction use *Berberis*, *Lycopodium*, *Phosphorus*, *Nux vomica* or *Chelidonium*. Refer to the relevant section of this book.

Where specific allergy is diagnosed, potentised *allergen* (e.g. House Dust, Fleas or Grasses) may be a helpful adjunct to constitutional therapy. Allergy is only a *symptom* of immune dysfunction.

For flea control a safer approach is to use essential oils. Should these fail, garlic and brewers yeast, fed to the dog or cat, may also produce a hostile environment for fleas. Flowers of Sulphur in the drinking water and homoeopathic *Sulphur* by mouth may also help. Flea collars can be obtained, containing only natural herbal or essential oil ingredients. Resort to chemicals should be very cautious and, if proven necessary, choice of chemical should lean toward the less hazardous preparations since some products do contain some very powerful modern chemicals (e.g. Organophosphorus compounds). Useful tips are provided in *Natural Remedies for Your Cat*, Piccadilly Press, by the same author.

Where Neoplasia exists, refer to section on Neoplasia p. 124.

Where dietary problems are suspected, the diet should be corrected. Homoeopathic potencies of the dietary minerals greatly help the animals to adjust its metabolism for that mineral (see p. 43).

In all cases a remedy to match the symptoms (see below) may be used (however if ectoparasites or ringworm are involved it may not be sufficient to rely on a homoeopathic remedy alone). *Always remember the constitutional approach since skin disease is a whole body disorder*.

'Symptomatic'* Treatment of Skin Disorders

The choice of remedy must, in the final instance, rest with one's knowledge of the materia medica of the remedies. Chapter 17 only provides

---

* This term is used in this text to imply selection of a homoeopathic medicine according to the symptoms displayed. This is only an aide-memoire and should not override 'constitutional' considerations to which the symptoms are often a pointer.

a very basic materia medica. For a wider knowledge of the remedies consult other works such as Clarke, Boericke, Kent or Tyler. Only by reading different authors can one begin to obtain a valuable working knowledge of remedies. The following are given as useful suggestions. *Constitutional principles are very important and should be an overriding consideration when prescribing.*

Allergic type swellings (Urticaria) (p. 119)	*Apis, Astacus, Bovista, Chamomilla, Medusa*, potentised *allergens, Pulex, Urtica*
Alopecia	*Alumen, Arsen. alb., Kali ars., Lycopodium, Nat. mur., Pix liquida, Selenium, Thallium, Ustilago*
Anal Adenomata	*Thuja*
Anal Glands	*Calendula* lotion, *Hepar sulph., Sanicula, Silica, Tarentula cub.*
Bends of limbs	*Aethusa, Ammonium carb., Ant. crud., Graphites, Kali arsen., Lycopodium, Nat. mur., Sepia*
Blackened skin	*Berberis, Kali arsen., Lachesis, Sepia, Sulphanilamide, Thuja*
Bruises	See Injury p. 123
Burns	See p. 120
Cracks/Fissures	*Ant. crud., Cistus, Graphites, Petroleum, Pix liquida*
Eyes (around)	*Chrysarobinum, Psorinum, Sulphur* (see also Allergic) (also p. 60)
Face/Chin area	*Ant. crud., Borax, Cicuta vir., Dulcamara, Graphites, Hepar sulph., Mezereum, Psorinum, Silica, Staph./Strep. nosodes, Sulphur, Sulph. iod.* (also p. 58)
Genital area	*Alumina, Ammon. carb., Caladium, Croton tig., Hydrastis, Picric acid, Sanicula*
Induration	(e.g. Lick Granuloma) *Calc. fluor., Ignatia, Silica, Tarentula cub., Thuja*
Interdigital Cysts	*Calc. sulph., Graphites, Hepar sulph., Lachesis, Silica*

Intertrigo	*Causticum, Graphites, Hepar sulph., Petroleum, Sulphur*
Itching	*Alumen, Alumina, Ammon. carb., Anacardium, Ant. crud., Arsen. alb., Bacillinum, Caladium, Calc. carb., Cistus, Dolichos, Graphites, Hypericum, Lycopodium, Mercurius, Mezereum, Nat. mur., Primula obcon., Psorinum, Pulsatilla, Rhus tox., Sepia, Sulphur, Sulph. iod., Urtica*
Labial folds	*Ant. crud., Arsen. alb., Causticum, Clematis, Condurango, Graphites*
Mucocutaneous Junction	*Condurango, Fluor. acid., Nit. acid, Sulphur*
Nail bed	*Hepar sulph., Myristica, Sarsap., Silica*
Nails	*Alumina, Calc. carb., Graph., Silica, Thuja*
Red, blotchy	*Arsen. alb., Belladonna, Cistus, Hypericum, Primula obc., Ranunculus bulb., Rhus tox., Urtica*
Ringworm (and circular patches in general)	*Bacillinum, Berberis, Chrysarobinum, Sepia, Tellurium*
Rodent Ulcer	See Mucocutaneous Junctions, also: *Asterias, Calendula* lotion, *Cistus can., Conium, Galium ap. Ø, Hydrastis, Mercurius, Nitric acid, Sulphur* (see also Mouth p. 73).
Scabs and Miliary Eczema	*Ant. crud., Calc. sulph., Dulcamara, Mezereum, Pulex, Rhus tox., Selenium* (p. 90)
Scaly	*Ant. crud., Arsen. alb., Kali sulph., Nat. mur., Psorinum, Rhus tox., Sulphur*
Scurf	*Arsen alb., Fluor. acid, Sepia, Sulphur, Thuja*
Sebaceous Cysts	*Baryta carb., Calc. sil., Calc. sulph., Conium, Kali iod.*
Sunburn (rare)	*Cantharis, Hypericum* lotion
Tail Eczema	*Calc. fluor., Mercurius, Tarentula cub.*

Thickened skin   *Hydrocotyle, Kali ars., Sulphanil., Thuja*
Vesicles   *Ant. crud., Rhus tox., Sulphur*
Weeping Eczema   *Cantharis, Croton tig., Graphites, Hepar*
                        sulph., Kreosotum, Mercurius, Myristica seb.
Warts   *Causticum, Nitric acid, Thuja**

GENERAL REMEDIES:

Ichthyolum   Is a good antiparasitic remedy.
Myristica seb.   Is a good skin disinfectant.

At all times bear in mind the total patient and think in terms of a constitutional remedy where possible, also keeping in mind the general notes at the start of the chapter (p. 56).

NERVOUS SYSTEM

This section will not attempt to discuss the mental problems of animals since those will be covered in Chapter 12. Some conditions of the Nervous System will be found in other sections, for example, Nerve injury, Concussion and Brain injury (p. 123); Disc lesions and ankylosing conditions of the spine (see Locomotor p. 100); Trembling and Paralysis will be found under muscles (p. 105); Eclampsia has been discussed on p. 94. Key Gaskell syndrome is on p. 134. Conditions not covered elsewhere are:

Tetanus is a specific disease of the nervous system leading to opisthotonus, lockjaw and death in severe cases! It is not unknown in dogs despite popular opinion. There is hypersensitivity to stimuli. The organism involved is Clostridium tetani which usually gains entrance via puncture wounds (pp. 130 and 124). Prognosis for dogs is good if treated homoeopathically in the early stages.

The specific *nosode* should be used in conjunction with *Angustura, Hypericum, Ledum, Stramonium* or *Strychninum* according to signs shown plus *Hydrocyanic acid* if there is cyanosis.

Opisthotonus without tetanus, which does occur on occasions as a

---

* A great many remedies have warts in their provings, so this is only a very short list.

result of injury or poisoning, should be treated by such remedies as *Cicuta, Ignatia, Nux vomica, Upas* or the above, chosen according to the symptoms showing and the cause.

Chorea describes the rhythmic unusual motion of head and other parts as a result of brain damage by such agents as Distemper virus. Where a specific agent is involved, the relevant *nosode* should be given. Other remedies of possible assistance are:

Agaricus, Cicuta vir., Conium, Hyoscyamus, Mygale, Stramonium, Strychinum

Convulsions and Fits (including Epilepsy). Epileptiform fits can take many forms (beware of heart attack differential diagnosis). Often a study of possible causes can be of more use than attempting to treat by symptoms. A paper is published in IJVH (see also p. 113 and p. 145).

Where teething may be involved	*Chamomilla*
Where roundworms may be involved	*Cina*
Where the animal misses its owner or member of the family or mate or a previous home (see Chapter 16).	*Ignatia*
Where temper seems to be involved	*Nux vomica*
Where male hypersexuality contributes	*Conium, Gelsemium, Picric acid*
Where excitability can overflow into epilepsy (see also 'excitability' later in this section)	*Ignatia, Mag. phos., Phosphorus, Zincum met.*
If fear is the cause	*Aconite*

Also effective are the following, according to symptoms and situations:

Agaricus, Belladonna, Calc. carb., Cicuta, Cocculus, Hyoscyamus, Mag. phos., Mygale, Silica, Stramonium, Sulphur, Tarentula hisp., Thuja

As a good working shortlist the following should be studied carefully:

Belladonna, Chamomilla, Gelsemium, Ignatia, Silica

Also such nosodes as *Distemperinum* and *Lyssin* should be borne in mind.

Such poisons as *Mercurius, Metaldehyde, Organophosphorus* and *Strychnine* should also be considered as possible causes or, in potency, as remedies. Vaccination should not be ruled out as an aetiological agent, particularly in Setters, Cavaliers, Labradors and Retrievers.

Hysteria and Excitability are possibly two levels of the same problem and are even likely to be less severe extensions of the problem of fits and convulsions (see also Hyperactivity, Hysteria (p. 146)). Consider:

Where there is anticipatory fear	*Gelsemium*
Where pain is involved	*Chamomilla*
Where bad temper is part of the condition	*Nux vomica*
Where fever may be causing the trouble	*Belladonna*
Where there is much restlessness	*Arsen. alb.*
Where hysteria is uppermost	*Hysocyamus, Stramonium, Veratrum album*

Passiflora, Scutellaria and *Valeriana* are all good 'sedating' remedies, as too are herbal Skullcap, Valerian, Hops, Passion flower.

Horner's Syndrome. This is characterised by unilateral (usually) loss of function of the muscles of the eyelids (the upper lid drops, the lower lid can be raised). There is usually constriction of the pupil on the affected side. It is involved with loss of function of some nerves, particularly the sympathetic nerves to the area. It is not analogous with the human stroke syndrome. There is overlap with the 'Canine stroke' syndrome referred to below. Remedies which may help are: *Aconite, Gelsemium, Morphinum, Physostigmine* or *Pilocarpus*. Spontaneous resolution can occur in some cases.

Loss of Balance (vertigo) as may happen in middle ear problems (see Ear p. 71) and brain damage, vestibular syndrome ('Canine stroke') and Horner's Syndrome (q.v.), anaesthesia etc. can be helped by:

Loss of balance on shaking head	*Conium*
Where concussion is involved	*Helleborus*

Vertigo from nervousness	*Argent. nit.*
With extreme sensitivity to noise	*Theridion*
As a result of heat stroke	*Glonoinium,*
	Lachesis
Vertigo of the aged animal especially after rest	*Phosphorus*
Falls to left, head rolls from side to side,	
choreic movements	*Zincum*
Falls to right	*Causticum*

Facial paralysis loss of function of the nerves to the facial muscles (usually unilateral) will result in distortion of the face. The ear, eyelids, lips and maybe also tongue are often affected. The distortion of the lips can lead to unilateral drooling and there may be a problem with swallowing, depending upon which nerve is affected. Useful remedies are:

Aconitum, Belladonna (R), *Causticum* (R), *Gelsemium, Senega* (L), *Verbascum* (L).

CDRM, particularly applying to German Shepherds, is a demyelinating condition and therefore is a disease of nerve malfunction and degeneration. It has been treated with *Causticum, Conium, Lathyrus* or *Plumbum met.*; but when advanced it is not easily treated. When caught in the early stages, results may be achieved in preventing development especially when acupuncture is used as an adjunct to homoeopathic treatment. Immune processes are implicated. This condition carries a very poor prognosis but paradoxically the outlook has been found to be slightly better in dogs which are older at time of onset, when treated holistically.

ENDOCRINE SYSTEM

The Endocrine System is a finely balanced and complex control mechanism for the reactions and metabolism of the body. The main glands are the Pituitary, Thyroid, Adrenal, Parathyroid and Pancreas (q.v.). The gonads also form part of the system but appear to be less critical for overall health. Problems associated with this system should respond to correct constitutional prescribing but may also require a more specific stimulus, using a potency of the appropriate *glandular tissue* or its *hormone*. Serious malfunction of the glands would require veterinary help and is beyond the scope of this book. As a general guide, low potency remedies of a specific gland stimulate that gland and high potencies suppress its activity.

SUMMARY

It has been stated many times in this book, simply because it is so fundamental to the principles of homoeopathy, that the foregoing pages of this chapter are a handy reference guide only. They are not, and cannot be, a full manual on the treatment of disease. Please use them freely but always with the consideration uppermost, that homoeopathy relies for a cure on the use of the principles laid down by Hahnemann in the following steps:

a) Know the remedies (a study of Materia Medica)
b) Know the disease (a study of the patient, i.e. the totality of symptoms).
c) Match a remedy to the disease in question taking all considerations into account.

And fourthly:

d) Remove any obstacles to recovery.

This last step includes a consideration of environmental and nutritional factors (so vital in farm animal medicine but also of immense importance in the correct management of small animal cases, see *Feeding Dogs the Natural Way* by the same author) and is as important as the preceding three steps if a real cure is to be obtained. See also pp. 14–16 and Chapters 4, 5, 6 and Appendix 8. It also includes any necessary supportive therapy (e.g. fluids and electrolytes).

CHAPTER 9

The Modalities

The modalities are the ways in which a symptom is affected by such factors as weather, time of day, movement, temperature, etc. These are ascertained by asking 'what makes the symptom better/worse?' A knowledge of some of these properties of the medicines will make prescribing easier and more effective. They may often be the strongest lead to the correct choice of remedy in a given case.

Aggravations (that is symptoms are made worse by)

Air – cold, dry:	*Aconite, Arsenicum, Bryonia, Psorinum, Rhododendron, Spongia*
Air – open:	*Aconite, Nux vomica*
Anger:	*Bryonia, Chamomilla, Nux vomica, Staphysagria*
Bright objects:	*Belladonna, Cantharis, Stramonium*
Cold:	*Aconite, Arsen. alb., Bryonia, Causticum, Chamomilla, Dulcamara, Hepar sulph., Mag. phos., Nux vomica, Rhododendron, Rhus tox., Sepia, Silica*
Cold Dampness:	*Calc. carb., Dulcamara, Mercurius, Rhus tox.*
Dampness:	*Calc. carb., Colchicum, Dulcamara, Rhus tox.*
Drinking:	*Arsen. alb., Cantharis, Mercurius, Rhus tox.*
Excitement:	*Aconite, Argent. nit., Coffea, Colchicum, Colocynth, Conium, Gelsemium, Hyosc., Ignatia, Nux vomica, Petroleum, Phosphorus*
Food – after:	*Argent. nit., Arsen. alb., Bryonia, Calc. carb., Carbo veg., Colchicum, Nux vomica, Pulsatilla, Sepia*

Fright: *Aconite, Ignatia*

Jarring: *Belladonna, Bryonia, Spigelia*

Light: *Belladonna, Conium, Merc. cor., Nux vomica, Phosphorus, Stramonium*

Lying down: *Arsen. alb., Belladonna, Conium, Phosphorus, Pulsatilla, Rhus tox.*

Movement: *Arnica, Baptisia, Belladonna, Borax, Bryonia, Cocculus, Petroleum, Phytolacca, Sanicula, Spigelia, Veratrum*

Noise: *Aconite, Belladonna, Coffea, Ignatia, Nux vomica, Theridion*

Overheating: *Aconite, Ant. crud., Belladonna, Bryonia, Glonoinium, Lachesis, Nux vomica*

Pressure: *Apis, Hepar sulph., Lachesis, Merc. cor.*

Rest: *Arnica, Arsen. alb., Merc. sol., Pulsatilla, Rhus tox., Ruta grav., Sepia*

Lying on R. side: *Belladonna, Bryonia, Causticum, Chelidonium, Lycopodium, Mag. phos., Mercurius*

Lying on L. side: *Bellis per., Colchicum, Colocynth, Lachesis, Lil. tig., Spigelia, Thuja*

Storm – before: *Bellis per., Nat. sulph., Rhododendron*

     – during: *Nat. carb., Phosphorus*

Swimming: *Ant. crud., Rhus tox., Sulphur*

Time

   – in morning: *Bryonia, Calc. carb., Kali bich., Lachesis, Nat. mur., Nux vomica, Phosphorus, Pulsatilla, Sulphur*

   – in afternoon: *Apis mell., Belladonna, Calc. carb., Colocynth, Hepar sulph., Lycopodium, Phosphorus, Pulsatilla*

   – in evening: *Aconite, Belladonna, Bryonia, Chamomilla, Lycopodium, Mercurius, Phosphorus, Pulsatilla, Rhus tox., Sepia*

   – at night: *Aconite, Arsen alb., Belladonna, Coffea, Drosera, Lachesis, Mercurius, Nit. acid, Pulsatilla, Rhus tox., Spongia, Sulphur*

Touch: *Aconite, Apis mel., Arnica, Belladonna, Bryonia, Chamomilla, Colchicum, Hepar sulph., Mag. phos., Nitric acid, Nux vomica, Plumbum, Silica, Strychninum*

Ameliorations (that is symptoms are made better by)

Air – open: *Allium, Alumina, Apis, Argent nit., Cinchona, Glonoinium, Lycopodium, Nat. mur., Pulsatilla, Sepia*

Back – arching: *Colocynth, Mag. phos.*

Being carried: *Chamomilla*

Cold: *Bryonia, Ledum, Phosphorus*

Cold application: *Apis, Belladonna, Phosphorus, Pulsatilla*

Cold water: *Bryonia, Phosphorus, Pulsatilla*

Consolation: *Chamomilla*

Damp weather: *Causticum*

Dark: *Euphrasia, Merc. cor.*

Exercise: *Rhus tox.*

Lying down: *Bryonia, Colchicum, Nat. mur., Pulsatilla*

Motion: *Alumina, Cyclamen, Dulcamara, Nitric acid, Rhus tox., Sepia*

Pressure: *Argent. nit., Bryonia, Chelidonium, Colocynth, Ignatia, Mag. phos., Pulsatilla, Sepia*

Rest: *Bryonia, Colchicum, Nux vomica*

Swimming: *Causticum*

Touch: *Bryonia, Calc. carb.*

Warmth: *Arsen. alb., Colocynth, Dulcamara, Hepar sulph., Ignatia, Mag. phos., Nux vom., Phos. acid, Psorinum, Rhus tox., Silica*

All these listings are to be taken as a guide only but can prove very useful in choosing between two remedies for a particular case. The author has not verified every one of them in animals but has included a few unverified remedies according to their reputation in human treatments. Beware 'false' modalities, eg. an evening modality may, in reality, be a post prandial modality, since a dog may be fed in the evening.

CHAPTER 10

The Generalities and First Aid Measures

This section is a 'quick prescribing' aide memoire for general conditions not covered under any previous section in this book.

In some parts of this section little guidance will be given for choice of remedy since reference to materia medica is important. In alphabetical order:

Allergy: Such remedies as *House dust* and *Grass pollens* are indicated in conditions arising from those allergies. *Galphimia glauca* is a non specific anti-allergic remedy. *Apis mell.*, *Ars. alb.*, *Astacus*, *Bovista*, *Fragaria*, *Primula obconica*, *Rhus tox.* and *Urtica* have all been used with varied success in allergic conditions according to symptoms and cause if found. Remember, this is a disturbance of immune function and constitutional prescribing may be the optimum route to follow.

Anaemia: Apart from standard veterinary supportive treatments consider:

Where red blood cells are damaged	*Chin. sulph.*, *Trinitrotulene*
Where debility after long illness is the factor	*Acetic acid.*, *China*, *Ferr, phos.*, *Phos. acid*
Where malnutrition is involved	*Calc. phos.*, *Ferrum met.*, *Silica*

When haemorrhage has preceded it	*Acetic acid* (dropsy), *Arsen. alb.* (restless)
When toxaemia has contributed	*Mercurius, Phosphorus*
From deficiency in haemopoiesis	*Cuprum, Ferrum ars., Plumbum*
Haemolytic with jaundice	*Lycopodium, Phos., Merc.*
Failure of clotting mechanism	*Crotalus, Lachesis, Melilotus, Phos., Secale*

Aphonia and Dysphonia (where the voice is lost or altered):

From too much barking	*Causticum, Collinsonia*
From hysteria	*Gelsemium*

Appetite (may be a symptom of serious disease, seek veterinary advice):

Variable	*Pulsatilla*
Voracious	*Abrotanum, Calc. carb., Calc. phos., Cina, Iodum*
Increased but quickly satisfied	*Lycopodium, Sepia*
Depraved	*Calc. carb., Calc. phos., Cina, Phosphorus*

Bites (cat or dog):   *Arnica, Hepar sulph., Calendula* lotion. The need for antibiotics is usually eliminated but, depending upon which site is injured, **veterinary attention** should be sought.

Bites and Stings (from insects):   *Apis, Arnica, Cantharis, Hypericum, Ledum, Urtica, Hypericum/Calendula* lotion or *Arnica* lotion

Bites (from snake):   *Cedron, Echinacea, Tarentula, Vipera* – **seek urgent veterinary attention.**

Burns/Scalds: *Apis mell., Arnica, Cantharis, Urtica,* Infected: *Hepar sulph.*

Collapse: *Carbo veg., Camphora, Laurocerasus* Ø, **seek urgent veterinary attention**.

Convalescence: *Acetic acid, Calc. carb., Calc. phos., China, Ferrum phos., Kali carb., Lecithin, Phos. acid*

Dehydration: *China, Phos. acid,* **seek veterinary advice**.

Fever: *Aconite, Belladonna, China, Chin. sulph., Echinacea, Gelsemium, Lachesis, Pulsatilla, Pyrogen, Sulphur* (**veterinary attention** may be necessary).

Frost Bite: *Agaricus.* If followed by:

Gangrene: *Carbo veg., Echinacea, Lachesis, Secale,* **seek veterinary attention**.

Haemorrhage: Treat homoeopathically according to the character of the blood and bleeding. **Veterinary attention** should be sought if any quantity of blood is being lost. See also post operative problems.

From trauma	*Arnica, Millefolium*
With coldness, convulsions etc.	*China*
Bright red	*Aconite, Ipecacuanha, Millefolium, Nitric acid*
Clotting with bright fluid	*Ferrum, Sabina*
Clotting dark	*Elaps, Hamamelis, Thlaspi*
Watery, dark, decomposing	*Crotalus, Lachesis, Secale*
Watery, bright	*Phosphorus*
Heavy breathing	*Ipecacuanha*
Anxiety	*Aconite*
Collapse	*Carbo veg.*
Active haemorrhage, bright red	*Nitric acid*

	Post operative seepage	*Strontia*
	Post partum, red flow	*Nitric acid, Sabina*
	Post partum, build up then gushes	*Ipecacuanha*
	Post partum, continual, dark	*Secale*
	After serious	*Acetic acid, Arsen.*
	haemorrhage consider	*alb., Phos. acid, Strontia*

Heat Stroke: *Belladonna, Gelsemium, Glonoinium, Natrum mur., Natrum sulph., Sulphur*

Hypersexuality: *Camphor, Conium, Lyssin, Picric acid, Pulsatilla* (see also pp. 87, 91, 146)

Ill Effects of (see also 'Never Well Since . . .' p. 125):

	Abortion	*Kali carb.*
	Anaesthetic	See post operative problems.
	Anxiety/Apprehension leading to:	
	Diarrhoea	*Arg. nit.*
	Incontinence	*Gelsemium*
	Restlessness	*Arsen. alb.*
	Near paralysis	*Gelsemium*
	Stupor	*Opium*
	Autumn and changeable weather	*Dulcamara*
	Chilling (p. 140)	*Aconite*
	Cold and Damp weather	*Dulcamara, Rhus tox.*
	Cold, dry weather	*Aconite, Rhododendron*
	Excitement	*Argent. nit., Coffea, Gelsemium*
	Grief	*Ignatia, Nat. mur., Phos. acid*
	Haemorrhage	see Haemorrhage
	Heat	*Glonoinium, Sulphur*
	Illness	see Convalescence.

Injury	*Arnica*
Over exertion	*Arnica, Phos. acid*
Over eating	*Nux vomica*
Parturition	*Caulophyllum, Pulsatilla, Sabina, Sepia* (see also Female p. 92)
Rotten food	*Arsen. alb., Camphor, Pyrogen, Veratrum album*
Shock	*Aconite, Arnica*
Specific diseases	See 'Never Well Since . . .' p. 125 and Specific Diseases p. 129.
Surgery	See Post Operative Problems p. 126.
Vaccination	*Ant. tart., Lach., Puls., Silica, Thuja* (also pp. 107, 158, 160)

Injury: Always *Arnica* then think of:

Adhesions:	*Calc. fluor, Silica*
Bone	*Ruta grav., Symphytum*
Brain/Head	*Baryta carb., Cicuta, Helleborus, Nat. sulph., Opium*
Bruising	*Arnica, Bellis per., Hamamelis*
Concussion	*Helleborus, Nat. sulph, Opium*
Cornea	*Ledum, Merc. cor.*
Extremities (rich in nerve endings)	*Hypericum*
Graze	*Arnica, Hypericum/ Calendula* lotion

Joints/Fibrous tissue	Rhus tox., Ruta grav.
Orbital area	Symphytum
Periosteum	Ruta grav.
Scar tissue breaking open	Causticum
With Shock/Fright	Aconite
Sphincters	Staphisagria
Spinal	Helleborus, Hypericum, Nux vomica
Deep Tissues (esp. Pelvic)	Bellis per.
Wounds	
Bleeding:	Phos., Strontia
Cuts:	Staphysagria, Calendula lotion
Granulation (exuberant):	Nitric acid, Silica, Thuja
Haematoma (ear):	Arnica, Hamamelis
Infected:	Hepar sulph., Calendula lotion
Laceration:	Arnica, Calendula lotion
Old injuries (won't heal):	Calc. sulph., Causticum, Graphites, Silica
Puncture:	Ledum
Scar tissue:	Calc. fluor., Graphites, Sil., Thuja, Thiosin.
Ulcerated/ Ungranulated:	Arsen alb., Galium aparine Ø
Neoplasia:* Any Malignancy	Arsen. alb., Viscum alb.
Abdominal	Hydrastis

* Neoplasia has been treated by the author with Iscador® therapy (anthroposophical) with varying results. More work needs to be done on this to increase predictability of results.

Bony	See Skeletal System p. 100, *Calc. fl.*, *Hekla lava*
Lipoma	*Baryta carb.*, *Thuja*
Lymphatic	See Lymphatic p. 99.
Mammary	See Female p. 96.
Stomach	*Hydrastis, Ornithogallum Ø* See Digestive System p. 77.
Ulcerated	*Asterias*
Warts	See Skin p. 111.

Always pay special attention to diet in cases of neoplasia. Although, statistically, results are not good, there have been many cases of recovery from malignant disease in dogs while under homoeopathic and holistic nutritional management. Remember constitutional prescribing.

'Never well since . . . ': This is in quotation marks since it is a common saying of both human patients and pet carers during history taking. It means what it says and can be followed by any of life's events (illness, specific disease, pregnancy, parturition, surgery, birth, oestrus, poisoning, vaccination, injury etc.). When such a sentence appears in the history one should not ignore it, it can be the key to the successful treatment of the case. Treat such historical comments as if they were part of the present symptoms and surprising results can follow. See Chapter 16 – Case Histories for examples. See also pp. 42, 122, 123.

Nystagmus: *Agaricus, Cicuta, Gelsemium, Physostigma,* according to concomitant symptoms.

Obesity: This is not really a disease state but can be helped by a) Male and Female treatment as per pp. 90 and 96, if applicable, b) *Calc. carb.*, *Capsicum, Graphites, Kali carb.*, according to symptoms, also *Phytolacca berry* Ø.

Photophobia: *Aconite, Argent. nit., Belladonna, Conium, Euphrasia, Mercurius, Rhus tox.*, according to concomitant symptoms (see also p. 64).

Post Operative Problems:

	Adhesions	*Acetic acid, Calc. fl.*
	Anaesthetic problems	potentised *Anaesthetic, Acetic acid, Nux vom., Opium*
	Bladder surgery	*Staphisagria*
	Bleeding	*Strontia* (and see Haemorrhage).
	Bone surgery	*Symphytum, Ruta grav.*
	Bruising	*Arnica,* (if deep bruising) *Bellis per., Symphytum*
	Constipation	*Nux vomica*
	Convalescence help	*Kali phos., Phos. acid, Phosphorus*
	Dental surgery	*Arnica, Hypericum, Ruta grav.*
	Eye surgery	*Senega, Symphytum*
	Fear	*Aconite*
	Gassy Colic	*China, Colocynth, Raphanus*
	Intestinal Stasis	*Carbo veg., Nux vomica, Opium*
	Joints	*Bryonia, Rhus tox., Ruta grav.*
	Oedema	*Apis mell.*

	Pain	
	Unwilling to move a muscle:	*Bryonia*
	General pain symptoms:	*Hypericum*
	Irritable pain:	*Chamomilla*
	Recovery slow, languid and shivery	*Kali sil.*
	Renal colic	*Berberis*
	Sepsis	*Hepar sulph.*, *Pyrogen* (see below).
	Shock (q.v.)	*Camphor, Strontia, Veratrum album*
	Soreness around wound	*Rhus tox., Staphisagria*
	Vomiting	*Ipecacuanha, Nux vomica, Phosphorus, Staphisagria*
	Always remember *Arnica* and *Calendula* wherever possible.	
Pre Operative:	Anxiety and fear (see pp. 144/145).	*Aconite, Argent nit.* or *Gelsemium*
	Bronchial problems	*Antimonium tart.*
	Bruising preventive	*Arnica*
	Heart therapy	See p. 98.
Sepsis and Abscess:	Acute	*Hepar sulph., Myristica sebifera*
	Chronic	*Calc. sulph., Silica*
	Dental Abscess	*Merc sol.*
	Embedded foreign body	*Silica*
	With local purpling	*Lachesis, Tarentula cub.*
	With Septicaemia	*Arsen. alb., Echinacea, Pyrogen*

| | With Toxaemia | *Arsen alb.,* |
| | | *Echinacea, Pyrogen* |

Hepar sulph. and *Merc. sol.* both tend to abort suppuration in low potency and encourage it in low potency.

Shock: *Aconite, Arnica, Camphor, Nat. mur., Veratrum album.* See also Post Operative p. 126. (*Bach Rescue Remedy*, although not homoeopathy, merits inclusion here).

Sleepless: *Apis mell., Arsen. alb., Chamomilla, Coffea, Nux vom., Pulsatilla, Scutellaria*

Terminal Illness: To ease sufferings prior to death or euthanasia* – *Arsen alb., Tarent. hisp.* or *cub.*

Thirst: Increased: *Aconite, Arsen alb., Bryonia, Calc. carb., Capsicum, Chamomilla, China, Lycopodium, Mercurius, Nat. mur., Phosphorus, Rhus tox., Veratrum album*
Increased thirst can herald serious disease so **consult a veterinarian** promptly and take a urine sample with you, collected in a clean, sterile pot.

Decreased: *Apis mell., Carbo veg., Gelsemium, Ignatia, Pulsatilla, Sabadilla*

Vaccinosis: See Chapter 15 and p. 123.

Weight Loss: *Acetic acid, Calc. phos., Glycerinum, Hydrastis, Iodum, Lecithin, Phos. acid, Silica, Thuja.* Seek **veterinary advice** since unexplained weight loss can be a sign of serious disease.

Worms: See p. 77.

Yawning: *Aconite, Chelidonium, Cocculus, Graphites, Ignatia, Lycopodium, Merc. cor., Platina, Sulphur.* This symptom often appears in a history taking and can, on occasions, be useful to help guide one to a remedy.

* The term euthanasia is used here, not because homoeopathic remedies will kill humanely but because they appear, when the body is *in extremis*, to remove the agony of indecision, bringing about either rapid and obvious restoration of the will to live or an easy passing

CHAPTER II

Specific Diseases

See also Chapter 14 – Prevention.

DOGS

Parvovirus Disease. This is a virus disease of repeated vomiting with bloody dysentery. Rapid dehydration and shock follow and collapse or death is very likely if treatment is ineffective.

Aconite as always is given in the very early stages.

Apormorphine, Arsen. alb., Phosphorus or *Veratrum album* are very useful to slow down or prevent the vomiting and diarrhoea. *Baptisia* has also been used on occasions. Be guided by presenting symptoms.

It is important to prevent the dehydration, both during and after the acute phase and here *China* or *Phos. acid* can be a great help in addition to fluid and electrolyte therapy. The *nosode* should also be given later, as in all specific diseases, to aid recovery. Homoeopathy has helped many cases to survive and recover.

Distemper/Hard Pad: This disease is not as common as it once was although in urban areas, where vaccination has not been universally accepted, it is still seen. It is a virus disease affecting all parts of the body including nervous system, digestive system, eyes, chest and skin. The nose and pads are frequently affected.

Aconite should be given, as usual, in the early febrile stages. The various symptoms, as they appear, should be treated according to the similia principle from knowledge of the Materia Medica. The sections on Eyes, Nervous system, etc. in Chapter 8 should be a guide to useful remedies.

Graphites, *Antimonium crud.*, *Nitric acid* and *Thuja* should be considered to help the involvement of the pads and nose. The *nosode* given later will help recovery.

Leptospirosis: This is a name encompassing disease associated with Leptospira icterohaemorrhagiae, which is associated mainly with liver disease and jaundice and Leptospira canicola which is associated mostly with kidney disease. The orthodox vaccination and proprietary homoeopathic *Leptospira nosode* include fractions relating to both organisms.

In the case of liver disease, *Phosphorus*, *Chelidonium*, *Berberis*, *Arsen alb.*, *Lycopodium*, *Mercurial* remedies and *Carduus mar.* should all be considered. *Aconite* should be given in the acute phase.

In the case of kidney involvement think of *Arsen. alb.*, *Berberis*, *Baptisia*, *Kali chlor.*, *Mercurius*, *Natrum mur.*, *Plumbum* and *Phosphorus* (see Kidneys).

The *combined nosode* should be used later, in either case, and continued after an apparent cure, in order to lessen the risk of 'carrier' status in surviving patients.

Hepatitis or Rubarth's Disease: This is rarely seen nowadays as a result of widespread conventional vaccination. It is a virus disease affecting mainly the liver but also all other parts of the body, since the virus is a virulent one. All mucous membranes are affected and kidney involvement gives rise to spread of disease. Coagulability of the blood is adversely affected and the eyes may become cloudy.

Aconite in the acute phase, as in all acute pyrexias, can be very beneficial. One then has to prescribe according to the prevalent symptoms at the time. See Throat, Mouth, Eyes, Liver, Kidneys and Haemorrhage for further details. In conjunction with 'symptomatic'* prescribing one should use the *Adenovirus nosode* later, to aid recovery and reduce the usually lengthy convalescent period. (* See footnote p. 132.)

Tetanus or Lockjaw: Arises from the toxin of the bacteria Clostridium tetani interfering with the neuromuscular junction. The result is an overstimulation of the muscles all over the body giving symptoms of jerking, hyperaesthesia, locked jaw (whence its name) and opisthotonus. The organism involved is anaerobic and favours puncture wounds for its proliferation. Hence the value of *Ledum* after puncture wounds. See Nervous System for treatments (p. 111). (Conventional vaccine is not routine although the disease is not unknown in dogs.)

Kennel Cough: This is probably associated with several organisms, among which are Bordetella and Parainfluenza. It is an upper respiratory tract infection but can rarely affect the lungs. It gains its name from the fact that it is able to spread most easily in boarding kennels where dogs are grouped together, so is most often seen after the summer holiday when a dog returns from boarding. Prevention is by use of the *nosode* and treatment is according to the guidelines on Coughs in Chapter 8. It is usually not a serious disease but can be very troublesome and annoying both, to dog and human companions, since the noise of the cough is very harsh and repeated frequently, the symptoms often lasting up to three weeks even with antibiotics. Conventional vaccine used not to be routine but it is usually now included in modern '7 in 1' vaccines (IJVH Vol. 2 No. 1, p. 45 and follow-up clarification article in Vol. 2 No. 2, p. 57). Correct homoeopathic prescribing will usually result in cessation of the cough within three days.

CATS

Panleucopaenia also known as **Feline Enteritis** and (mistakenly) as **Cat 'flu** (see later): This is a highly contagious and often fatal virus disease. Orthodox vaccination has reduced its incidence to a great extent but it is still seen in kittens and unvaccinated cats. Fever (where *Aconite*, as usual in the acute phase, can be useful), diarrhoea and severe dehydration characterise the disease.

Arsenicum, China, Echinacea, Mercurius and *Phos. acid* can all be of value depending on the symptoms (see Diarrhoea, etc.). Therapy in the form of fluid and electrolyte infusion is of great value also and should not be forgotten. Readers should be urged not to forget, when embarking on homoeopathy, the value of good, sound nursing and supportive therapy. Also remember the *nosode* later.

Cat 'flu or Feline Influenza: As in the human, is a complex condition associated with many viruses and secondary bacteria. Conventional vaccination may be of help but often viruses not included in the vaccine package can be involved, so prevention is not assured. The *nosode* or even a *specific nosode* for the outbreak, can be of great value in treatment and prevention and 'symptomatic'* treatment is invaluable. See Nose, Eyes, Throat, Sinuses etc. Dehydration owing to loss of appetite may also play a part, so remember *Phos. acid* or *China* and conventional fluid therapy if rehydration becomes vital.

Feline Infectious Anaemia: This is a malaria-like disease of the red blood cells (an over-simplified description). As with all infectious diseases, early fever can be helped with *Aconite* and a *nosode* could be used. Anaemia is the strong feature of the disease more than the febrile signs and here one should consider all remedies which are of help with anaemia, taking into account the concomitant symptoms (see Anaemia p. 119). *China* is an important remedy to consider. Remember supportive therapy, nutrition and vitamin and mineral treatment to aid recovery and blood regeneration, plus *Ferr., phos.*

Feline Infectious Peritonitis: This is an obscure viral disease causing gradual but extreme swelling of the abdomen with straw coloured fluid. Inappetance, jaundice, dyspnoea and weight lost can all be present. There are often white flecks in the abdominal fluid and white deposits on the peritoneal lining. A 'dry' form exists, in which symptoms usually centre on the chest. Use of the *nosode* will aid the recovery and elimination of virus. Symptomatic* treatment such as *Acetic acid, Apis mell., Blatta amer., Helleborus, Lycopodium, Tub. bov.* and *Senecio* are worth pursuing but the outlook is not good unless the case is caught early. Again, supportive treatment in the form of

---

* This term is used in this text to imply selection of a homoeopathic medicine according to the symptoms displayed. 'Constitutional' considerations should still apply, to which the symptoms will be a pointer.

fluids and electrolytes may be essential. A *nosode* is available to aid in prevention. The author sees many cases in a year and his own cats, protected by the *nosode*, have never contracted the disease during twenty-five years of practice, although often in contact with actively infective cases. In-contact cats in infected colonies have been given the homoeopathic preventive and cases have ceased. Also, most of those showing a positive blood test, but symptom-free at the time, seem to lose their positive titre over a period when regularly dosed. These comments are all applicable to FeLV and FIV too.

Feline Leukaemia (FeLV): This is a virus disease of the bone marrow, lymph nodes, lymphatic system in general, kidneys, immune system and haemopoietic system. Some cats will successfully recover under homoeopathic therapy but the outlook is not good unless cases are caught early. Supportive therapy, possible *nosode* therapy and 'symptomatic'* treatment are, again, the lines of treatment as in all infectious diseases (see also Lymphatic System p. 99 for remedies which may help.

Nosode preventive techniques are available and the same comments on efficacy of prevention and therapy apply as in Feline Infectious Peritonitis above. A conventional vaccine has recently come on the market but the author is cautious about this development.

Feline Immunodeficiency Virus (FIV): This infectious disease, once confused with Feline Leukaemia, is potentially lethal over a period, having similarities in action to HIV. However, preventive homoeopathic methods are available (same comments on efficacy as above under Feline Infectious Peritonitis) and many cases have survived well under homoeopathic therapy.

Chlamydia has recently been found to constitute an infectious disease in cats in its own right, bringing about respiratory and ocular symptoms. It is not unlike Feline Influenza in some of its manifestations. As with Feline Influenza, remedies can be selected according to

---

* This term is used in this text to imply selection of a homoeopathic medicine according to the symptoms displayed. 'Constitutional' considerations should still apply, to which the symptoms will be a pointer.

constitutional type and symptoms shown and the *nosode* can help in treatment or prevention in in-contacts.

Key Gaskell Syndrome (Feline Dysautonomia): This is a disease of unknown aetiology at present and was of very recent incidence at the time of the first edition. It seems to have more or less disappeared in the intervening years. It is included in this section on specific diseases (where one would expect to find diseases as a result of infection with specific organisms) because it caused a lot of worry and much mortality in the few years after it appeared and was first recognised. The outlook was not good but there were quite a number of successful recoveries, usually as a result of painstaking supportive therapy and nursing in conjunction with homoeopathy. As its alternative name suggests it is a disease affecting the autonomic nervous system. It is characterised by dilated pupils of the eye, dry mouth, malfunctioning bowels, difficulty in swallowing and gross dehydration. Supportive therapy is vital but several homoeopathic remedies exist which can be of help. Here again one has to choose between them on the basis of symptom matching (the similia principle).

Belladonna, *Calc. carb.*, *Gelsemium*, *Hyoscyamus*, *Nux moschata* and *Stramonium* are the ones used most often during the outbreak. One must consider primarily the mental disposition, as far as it can be determined, in prescribing a remedy but also take into account bowel function, abdominal distension, vomiting, etc. where signs are present. Other remedies used include *Alumina*, *Collinsonia*, *Lobelia*, *Nicotine*, *Neostigmine* and *Wyethia* (see also p. 67).

Salmonellosis: Salmonella can affect cats, guinea pigs, rabbits and mice and is usually characterised by a septicaemia and enteritis (often bleeding) resulting in very rapid death. It is preventable by the use of the *nosode* and *Baptisia* has a reputation in the control and cure of Salmonella disease. Treatment by *nosode*, *Baptisia* and appropriate similium should be successful if cases are caught in time. Here, again, appropriate use of antibiotic may 'buy' time if in doubt. Dogs appear to be very resistant to this disease, consistent with their evolutionary adaptation to scavenging. If raw meat (especially chicken) is offered to cats it should be organic, which will lessen the risk of Salmonella contamination.

RABBITS

Myxomatosis: A virus disease transmitted by rabbit flea infestation from the wild rabbit population. There is an orthodox vaccine available and there is also a homoeopathic preventive *nosode* as in the case of most specific diseases. This disease is characterised by a swollen head and neck (gelatinous tumours and fluid collect beneath the skin) and purulent ocular discharge. Loss of appetite, weakness and, eventually, death follow. Prevention is the key to this disease by use of the *nosode*. Treatment is often unsuccessful, the domestic rabbit being particularly susceptible to the disease. One should consider *Acetic acid, Abrotanum, Kali iod.* and *Mercurius sol.* for example, along with supportive therapy but the humanitarian justifications of persisting with a rabbit which is so ill with a poor prognosis are doubtful.

This discussion of a rabbit disease conveniently leads us on to a consideration of the particular problems to be found in the **smaller pets such as rabbits (lagomorphs), rodents, birds, reptiles, amphibians and fish**. It is essential to remember several points in connection with these species. Firstly, and this applies especially to the very small species, *they do not tolerate rough handling* and unless they are accustomed to handling by their carer, even the minimum can upset them badly.* Secondly, they are also very susceptible to **hypothermia,**† especially when ill, and care should be taken to ensure that this is not a problem. Thirdly, there are a number of idiosyncratic responses to conventional antibiotic therapy which consideration makes homoeopathy a very desirable and acceptable mode of treatment for these small and vulnerable creatures. Such idiosyncrasies are summarised by the following fatal incompatibilities:–

Guinea Pigs	Penicillin, Streptomycin and Erythromycin.
Hamsters	Penicillin, Streptomycin.
Birds	Streptomycin, Procaine Penicillin.

* Treat as for shock p. 128.   † See Chilling p. 122 and p 140

Fourthly, the nutrient requirements of these pets vary greatly and great care should be taken to ensure the correct diet for the species. Advice should be sought on this subject from someone properly experienced in the particular species. For example Guinea Pigs require Vitamin C in their diet when many other species do not, simply making their own in the bowel.

Fifthly, the management and housing of each species is very important and should be related to its own special biology. Care should be taken to seek reliable advice on this subject too.

Sixthly, just because these species are labelled 'exotics' it does not remove the need for a thorough examination and history taking, in so far as sympathetic handling can allow. A great many cases can only be solved via a proper clinical diagnosis and assessment and these can only be attained by attention to detail.

Where specific problems are covered in this text, reference to remedies should be used as a guide only. There is no substitute for homoeopathic prescribing by first principles, whatever the species. Bearing in mind the difficulties and dangers involved in handling some of these species, it is worth noting that homoeopathic remedies can be administered via the drinking water if the animal is not too ill to drink.

Diarrhoea in the Rabbit: is not a specific disease but it is worth considering here as a special subject. Often it can result from changes of diet, chilling, shock, milk feeding (rabbits unfortunately do like milk but it is a wholly unsuitable food) and it can also result from over-enthusiastic cleaning out of the droppings. In order to digest cellulose sufficiently some of the food passes twice through the digestive system and the rabbit produces two kinds of pellet. The crumbly pale green ones are those which have been through once and the dark shiny ones are the final product. The rabbit must be given access to the first stage droppings or digestive disorders can result and often a vitamin deficiency too, unless the diet has been formulated to obviate the need for this. Should diarrhoea occur, then treatment according to symptoms is important but consider especially *Colchicum* and *Mercurius*. **Coccidiososis** is a particularly virulent form of diarrhoea. For this a *nosode* and *Arsenicum* or *Mercurius* should help. One should consider also *China* or *Phos. acid* in cases of debility. Reference to major 'diarrhoea' remedies, however, is preferable to just picking on one or two likely remedies from this page (see p. 81 et seq).

Conjunctivitis and Rhinitis: are not uncommon where many rabbits are kept together but there are no special considerations applying to the rabbit. Refer to the pages on Eyes and Nose in Chapter 8.

Loss of Balance: is relatively common in the domestic rabbit and usually results from an ear infection. Consider *Conium, Hepar sulph.* and *Merc. sol.* as homoeopathic treatments and, if ear mites are involved, the infestation should be removed (see pp. 69 and 70). Essential oils may achieve this without the use of either insecticidal/acaricidal chemicals or compound proprietary drops which often contain steroids.

Salmonella: See Cats (p. 134).

Abscess: Rabbits can suffer from multiple abscesses, often associated with Pasteurella infection. This condition is potentially lethal and very difficult to treat. The *Myxomatosis nosode* may help and treatment with homoeopathic *Mercurius, Echinacea, Pasteurella nosode, Silica* or *Kali iod.* as appropriate will increase the chances of survival.

Tooth Problems: These usually only result from dietary imbalances, particularly with reference to calcium levels. If only the incisors are involved, they simply need clipping to keep them comfortable. If the cheek teeth are involved, then sadly anaesthesia and surgical intervention will probably be required. *Calc. phos.* or *Calc. fluor.* may help.

GUINEA PIGS

This species is very prone to **skin disorders** usually resulting from a deficiency of vitamin C but also a result of mange infection. Consider any symptom-based prescription but remember especially *Ant. crud., Graphites, Muriatic acid, Nat. mur., Phosphorus, Psorinum, Sulphur* and *Zincum met.*

Diarrhoea can also affect guinea pigs as in all other species and the remedies one should choose will be decided by the same factors (see p. 81 et seq).

Salmonella: See Cats (p. 134).

Tooth Problems: as for rabbits but much rarer, happily.

Handling and Management: see p. 135 et seq.

HAMSTERS

Dermatitis: Occurs in hamsters as in other species and choosing a remedy by symptoms and modalities is again the only way in which one can function. An exception to this would be the use of *Ignatia* or *Aconite,* should the appropriate circumstances have occurred to initiate the mental processes of bereavement or shock to which these little creatures can be especially prone. Remember *Rescue Remedy* too.

Wet Tail: This syndrome is not a specific disease but describes the appearance of the hamster with diarrhoea. Choose appropriate remedies by the usual homoeopathic means. The expected survival time of one of these tiny creatures, when affected with diarrhoea, is minimal so prompt action and good nursing are essential (see p. 81). *E. coli nosode* is a useful adjunct to appropriate homoeopathic medicines.

Handling and Management: see p. 135 et seq.

RATS AND MICE

These rodents suffer few diseases that are worthy of special mention but one which deserves a few lines is **Ringtail** in rats. Should the temperature and humidity in the environment be hostile, a disturbance of the blood circulation of the tail occurs and annular constrictions appear. The tail can drop off. A homoeopathic remedy which should be particularly effective here is *Secale*. Sadly though, once the condition has been noticed, it is often too late to prevent the consequences. For other problems the general discussions on other species apply.

Handling and Management: see p. 135 et seq.

CHINCHILLAS

It has been my pleasure over the years to be asked to treat a number of these congenial creatures in several different homes. Apart from problems all species suffer, many of their health difficulties stem from dietary, climatic and environmental differences between their natural home high in the Andes and our UK situation. Expert advice is needed to ensure correct conditions of diet and housing. Humidity is one such problem and **respiratory disease** can follow. Remedies to consider are *Dulcamara, Nat. sulph., Aranea, Thuja* and *Colchicum*. Beware moulds in dried forages. Constitutionally, many individuals fit the *Calcarea carbonica* picture but we also see **digestion problems** related to (for example) *Nux vomica*. However, no species can be entirely classified according to only one or two constitutional remedy pictures. As in rabbits, **tooth growth and wear** may cause problems but, if this happens, there is really only an anaesthetic and surgical option to try to correct abnormalities unless the problem is only in the incisor teeth. Such abnormalities will usually only result from incorrect diet, especially with regard to Calcium balance. *Calc. fluor.* may help.

Handling and Management: see p. 135 et seq.

BIRDS

By far the most common problem of birds brought to the veterinarian is **injury**. *Arnica, Rhus tox., Ruta grav.* and *Symphytum* are all equally as valuable to birds as they are to mammals. **Fracture** healing is aided by *Symphytum*, bruising is reduced by *Arnica* etc. Remember *Rescue Remedy*.

Aconite, *Hepar sulph.* and *Hypericum* are also used in their usual contexts and *Secale* can be of especial use in toe, leg and wing injuries, as circulation so often suffers. *Calendula* lotion is also of its customary value in the treatment of **wounds** so it is worth remembering homoeopathy can form as useful a form of first aid and continuing treatment in birds as in mammals.

Diarrhoea: see p. 81.

Mange: *Sulphur* is very useful and, in the particular problem in the budgerigar, of mange around the cere, consider in addition *Nitric acid*, *Silica* or *Thuja*, with *Hypericum/Calendula* lotion.

Eyes: No special notes, see section on Eyes p. 60.

Eggbound: Consider as a first treatment, *Caulophyllum* and *Sepia*. Use *Arnica* afterwards. Eggbinding may often result from an imbalance in calcium metabolism, causing eggshell abnormalities and poor tone in the oviducts and *Calcarea phos.* may help this. Consider also *Sepia* or *Helonias*.

Newcastle Disease, Paramyxo virus, Mycoplasmosis, Salmonellosis, Chlamydia (psittacosis) and other specific diseases should all be preventable by judicious use of the relevant *nosode* or treatable by the *nosode* and relevant 'symptomatic'* prescribing as outlined in the previous sections. The author has personal experience of treating some of these specific problems and sees no reason why the usual principles should not apply in others. Remember any Ministry of Agriculture regulations.

In the particular case of **Frounce** in pigeons consider *Graphites*, *Nitric acid* or *Rhux tox.* If lesions involve the **angles of the mouth** consider *Condurango*.

Feather Pecking: This very often results from mental disturbance (see p. 144). Consider also *Folliculinum, Sepia, Sulphur, Thallium.*

Chilling: *Aconite, Calc. carb., Calc. phos., Dulcamara, Rhus tox., Silica* (see also p. 122).

Handling and Management: see p. 135 et seq.

---

* This term is used in this text to imply selection of a homoeopathic medicine according to the symptoms displayed. 'Constitutional' considerations should still apply

TORTOISES, SNAKES, LIZARDS AND FISH

Poikilotherms are those animals which do not maintain their own body temperature but are totally at the mercy of the external environmental temperature. They are commonly called 'cold-blooded' but that is a relative term. Their body temperature can be high but only when the surroundings are very warm or when they bask in the sun.

Species commonly encountered in veterinary work are **Tortoises** (which hibernate) and their relatives, **Snakes**, **Lizards** and **Fish**. Homoeopathic work with these creatures is mainly confined to local or pathological prescribing (according to the same principles discussed for other species) as and when individual illnesses arise but an attempt can be made to aim for constitutional remedies in certain cases.

I am always reminded, when discussing these creatures, of the **Monitor Lizard** (a 'small' carnivorous iguana) which was constipated, off food and malevolently angry. He was also highly reactive to noise and disturbance. This was *Nux vomica* if ever I saw it and a single injection of *Nux* sorted the problem very rapidly!

Cleo the **Reticulated Python** was presented to me 'vomiting' blood and lethargic. She was also periodically thrashing with obvious abdominal discomfort. She had lost interest in her surroundings. She had last been fed two weeks earlier. It transpired that her environment was too cool (the species is indigenous to tropical rain forest) and I assumed she was suffering chilling, with her food not being digested properly, resulting in some putrefaction. I gave *Phosphorus 30c* by injection, according to 'constitutional' prescription, and *Pyrogenium* in low potency. Cleo had started to recover by the next evening.

A **Tortoise** was brought in suffering from respiratory problems. She was off food and had a right-sided conjunctivitis. *Lycopodium* was the treatment of choice and a good outcome ensued. *Lycopodium* appears to suit the tortoise appearance very well, as too can *Causticum hahnemannii*. Eggbound tortoises will respond very well to *Caulophyllum* usually within twenty-four hours.

The **Fish** which I have treated have been treated more according to 'herd' principles, which I have discussed in my book on cattle medicine, but individuals may also be treated. I have not knowingly prescribed 'constitutionally' for these creatures as I have established no feel for fish constitutional manifestations. Treatment has been by *nosodes* or by local/pathological methods only. This differs in no way from mammalian medicine, when practised on the same principles, but 'in water' treatment takes on a new meaning!

Handling and Management: see p. 135 et seq.

SUMMARY

Inevitably the author's experience with all the 'exotic species of pets is smaller than that with cats and dogs but results have been very encouraging and the foregoing pages should act as a guide to those intending to try homoeopathy on them.

In general terms, speed of response to remedies seems, in practice, to be governed more by life-style and general reactivity than body temperature. Horses and cats react very quickly to life's stimuli and so too to homoeopathic treatment. Tortoises react slowly, the Monitor Lizard reacted very quickly both in life-style and medically, as did the python. Do not be afraid to apply homoeopathic principles to these 'exotic' species, just because they are unusual visitors to the veterinary clinic. They are able to respond according to identical principles to those learnt for dogs and cats.

As always with homoeopathy, one can be assured of no harmful consequences arising out of its use. This holds true so long as, while trying to improve one's skills in the field of homoeopathy, one is not neglecting a perfectly good orthodox treatment or essential and well proven nursing procedure, to the detriment of the patient.

CHAPTER 12

Mental Problems

The scope of this book, and the obvious problems concerned with discerning mental symptoms in animals, precludes me from making this a lengthy chapter. Suffice to say that mental disorders most definitely do occur in pet animals and that one can sometimes discern them from the symptoms and behaviour shown and other times only divine them from circumstance. Many of the symptoms of such disorder are subjective and therefore locked within the patient, never to be observed by us. Some are objective, that is one can perceive them. It is the observation of behaviour which is of first importance, one has to evaluate it and then one has to deduce, if one can, what is the mental process governing it. It is at this stage that one can come adrift but it is always worth making the effort. A distinction should be made here between mental problems and those mental symptoms which are a part of any illness. There is, of course, overlap between these areas and a line of demarcation is not constructive and in fact cannot be drawn. The information contained in this chapter is mainly aimed at clear cases of mental disorder but the remedies mentioned can act as a useful aide memoire for use in other disorders in which mental symptoms are clear and discernible.

Mental problems can usefully be divided into three categories:–

1 Those whose symptoms are easily perceived from which one can relatively certainly deduce the underlying mental cause.
2 Those whose symptoms are not easily seen but the patient's demeanour betrays a mental problem whose nature may be very difficult to define.

3 Those whose symptoms appear as an entirely different manifestation in another organ, e.g. the skin or digestive system, and therefore may lead one to overlook the underlying mental cause, unsuccessfully attacking the visible clinical problem.

Go back to Hahnemann to remind yourself of the importance of all mental symptoms (remember he did have the advantage of access to subjective symptoms). Paras 210–213 inclusive, of Hahnemann's Organon draw one's attention to this concept. Refer to British Homoeopathic Journal Volume 73 No. 7 July 1983 page 165 for discussion of this problem when dealing with animals.

Demeanour and disposition will, of course, at all times affect one's choice of remedy in illness, especially in the constitutional context. However, there follows a list of remedies often associated with certain mental processes and it can act as a good guide in treating cases where one considers mental problems to be the major problem. The indications can also act as a guide to selection of a deeper constitutional remedy. Remember also the importance of treating historical problems (see p. 125 under 'Never Well Since . . . ') because an incident can leave a mental mark which, if untreated, can remain for a lifetime with a persistent effect on overall health.

Aggression	*Belladonna, Lycopodium, Nux vomica*
Anger	*Chamomilla, Colocynth, Crocus, Hepar sulph., Nux vomica*
Anxiety/ Apprehension	*Argent nit., Gelsemium, Lycopodium, Bach Rescue Remedy*
Aversions to:	
Being left	*Capsicum, Ignatia, Phosphorus, Phos. acid, Pulsatilla* (see also Bereavement/Loneliness and Fear of solitude).
Heat	*Sulphur*
Veterinary premises	*Argentum nit., Gelsemium, Lycopodium, Silica*
Bereavement/ Loneliness	*Aurum, Ignatia, Phos. acid, Psorinum, Pulsatilla*, (see also Aversion to being left and Fear of solitude).

Boredom	*Argent. nit., Arsen. alb., Lilium tigrinum, Lycopodium* (Boredom can lead to aimless activity including self-mutilation, see p. 109 Lick granuloma and p. 140).
Coprophagy	*Veratrum alb.*
Depraved appetite	*Calc. carb., Calc. phos., Cicuta, Cina, Cinchona, Cobaltum, Phosphorus*
Desires:	
Cold Water	*Arsen. alb., Bryonia, Mercurius, Pulsatilla*
Company	*Argent. nit., Arsen. alb., Lycopodium, Phosphorus*
Consolation/	
Reassurance	*Chamomilla, Pulsatilla*
Cool	*Sulphur*
Fresh Air	*Apis*
Heat	*Arsenicum, Psorinum*
Excitability	*Belladonna, Hyoscyamus, Ignatia, Mag. phos., Pulsatilla, Stramonium*
Fear/Fright/Shock	*Aconite, Nat. mur, Rescue Remedy*
Fear of:	
Being carried	*Borax, Sanicula*
Car	*Borax, Bryonia, Cocculus, Gelsemium, Sanicula*
Dark	*Phosphorus, Stramonium*
Forthcoming ordeal	*Argent. nit., Gels., Lycopodium, Silica*
Motion	*Bryonia*
Noise	*Nux vom., Phosphorus*
Solitude	*Hyosc., Kali carb., Lycopodium, Phos., Stramonium* (See also Aversion to being left and Bereavement/Loneliness).
Touch	*Arnica, Chamomilla, Lachesis, Nux vom., Plumbum* (abdomen).
Thunder	*Aconite, Borax, Gels., Hyosc., Nat. carb., Nat. mur., Phos., Rhododendron, Theridion*
Hyperactivity	*Arsen. alb., Coffea, Ignatia* (See also Excitability, Hysteria, Fits).

Hypersexuality	*Cantharis, Ferula, Gels., Hyosc., Origanum, Phos., Picric acid, Tarent. hisp.* (see also Sexual Systems and p. 122).
Hysteria	*Gels., Hyosc., Ignatia, Tarent. hisp., Valeriana* (see also Fits, pp. 112/113, Excitability, Hyperactivity).
Indifference	*Platina, Sepia*
Irritability	*Capsicum, Chamomilla, Cina, Crocus, Nux vom., Sepia*
Jealousy	*Apis mell., Lachesis*
Obstinacy	*Calc. carb., Silica, Sulphur, Tub. bov.*
Panic	*Aconite, Gels., Phos., Stramonium, Rescue Remedy*
Rage	*Hyoscyamus, Stramonium*
Resentment	*Lachesis, Staphisagria*
Restlessness/ Fidgeting	*Aconite, Arsen. alb., Chamomilla, Coffea, Ignatia, Rhus tox., Stramonium*
Roaming tendency	*Bryonia, Sulphur, Veratrum alb* (see also Hypersexuality).
Shyness/Timidity	*Baryta carb., Ignatia, Natrum mur., Pulsatilla, Silica, Sulphur*
Urination inappropriate (Spraying)	*Cantharis, Natrum mur., Staphisagria*

In all cases these suggestions can only be taken as a guide but this aide memoire can often give insight into a deep constitutional prescription or, at a lesser level, it may help to alleviate the worst behavioural traits when they become a problem.

CHAPTER 13

Special Problems of the Young and Old

Problems common in the adolescent male and female have been discussed at length under the heading of the Male and Female Sexual Systems – Chapter 8. It is worth considering separately however the particular problems of the very young and very old cat or dog to help bring what is written in earlier chapters into a practical context for these special patients.

PUPPIES/KITTENS THROUGH TO PUBERTY

Proper attention to the mother before, during and after the birth process is essential to the offspring's well being. Apart from all the benefit of proper nursing and management, study again the homoeopathic treatments outlined on p. 92 et seq. which have a particular benefit at this time. As for the offspring themselves, the results of a **traumatic birth** can be minimised with the use of *Arnica* (bruising), *Baryta carb.* and *Nat. sulph.* (brain damage), *Laurocerasus* (cyanosis) and *Aspidosperma* (respiratory failure). See also p. 93. Avoid all use of chemical drugs and vaccines in pregnancy in case of damage to the foetus and its healthy development. Homoeopathy, however, is a very useful and safe therapy during pregnancy and treating the mother will inevitably improve the lot of the foetus.

In the **suckling period** various problems can show themselves. **'Fading puppies'** is a condition manifesting itself in progressive loss of weight, strength and body temperature in newborn pups up to about three weeks of age. Hepatitis virus, Herpes virus, Escherichia coli and many other infective agents have been associated with this problem.

The progressive weakness leads to inability to suck and, commonly, death. There may or may not be diarrhoea. This condition is usually not encountered in the occasionally-bred dam on its own in a household but more commonly in larger breeding establishments where reservoirs of infection are built up. If the specific agent involved is known, then preventive measures during pregnancy and at birth should be adopted using the relevant homoeopathic *nosode*. Use *Aconite* in the early stages, *Arsenicum album*, if vomiting and diarrhoea are present, *Carbo veg.* if pups are cold and collapsed and *Abrotanum* if the navel is weeping. *Calc. phos.*, *China*, *Echinacea* and *Phos. acid* can all be of use according to the symptoms. The puppies should also be kept warm and dry with clean bedding. A hot water bottle insulated by three or four layers of towel (to prevent burning) is a good form of heating. Supportive fluid therapy may be valuable.

Diarrhoea in the very young should be treated according to symptoms as in all animals (see p. 81).

Kittens can have very **gummed up eyes** with cat 'flu virus infection and here the *nosode* can be of great use (as also in preventing the condition) in conjunction with such remedies as *Argent. nit.*, *Graphites* and *Pulsatilla*.

At a few days of age **dew claws** are often removed from puppies and in some breeds tails are still **docked**. *Aconite*, *Arnica*, *Hypericum* and *Staphisagria* are worth remembering for troubles at this stage.

When it comes to **weaning time**, *Ignatia* can prove useful for both dam and offspring, as too can *Phos. acid*, particularly if diarrhoea ensues. Both before and after weaning, pups can suffer from colic and even fits as a result of **round worm** infection. Here *Cina* or *Abrotanum* can be of tremendous value (p. 77).

Next is the period of **fast growth**, particularly for puppies, and here *Calc. fluor.* or *Calc. phos.* (according to constitution) should be remembered for adequate bone growth. One dose weekly for one or two months as a routine can be very beneficial.* **Diarrhoea** and **Colic** can be fairly common during the growing phase and should be treated according to symptoms (see Diarrhoea p. 81, Colic p. 78).

* See also pp. 43 and 100.

Teething can also cause many problems in this period and *Chamomilla* should always be borne in mind. Many cases of epileptiform fits arise from teething troubles and *Chamomilla* can stop this type of fit quite readily. Teething can cause many seemingly unrelated problems such as sore eyes, colic and diarrhoea too. Even some really persistent 'chewers' can be stopped with *Chamomilla*.

Insussusception, Hiccough, Foreign Body swallowing and **Travel Sickness** primarily occur in the young and growing pet and should be treated according to pp. 77 and 78.

Congenital heart problems and joint troubles also manifest themselves as the animal gains in weight and is moving towards full growth (these problems are discussed on pp. 100 and 102). Vaccination may be involved. **Entropion** also manifests itself as the puppy grows and a discussion of this problem is to be found on p. 62.

Vaccination is usually carried out between two and four months of age, if conventional vaccine is used, and this is not to be lightly decried since it has saved countless dogs from the more terrible effects of Distemper, Hepatitis, Parvovirus and Leptospirosis. Homoeopathic prevention of these diseases by the *nosode* can be instituted at an earlier age, however, as also for Enteritis, 'flu and other virus diseases for kittens (see Chapters 11, 14). Many use the *nosodes* alone, but they can also be used alongside conventional vaccination. Should any harmful effects of conventional vaccine be experienced, the relevant *nosodes* should be given along with *Thuja* or appropriate constitutional remedy. On occasions too, the adjuvant portion of a killed vaccine can cause trouble (e.g. Aluminium Hydroxide) whereupon the potentised (homoeopathic) form of this can be given with great effect, reducing the local pain, general symptoms and risk of abscessation. Because of some of the problems associated with modern conventional vaccination, a great many people do not use these agents but turn to homoeopathic *nosodes* instead, for the protection of their feline and canine charges (see p. 158 for a fuller discussion of this issue). This practice has been going on for a great many years but only now is being openly discussed in the press. The author uses only this method for his own pets, horses and family.

Towards the end of the growing period in dogs, **puberty** starts to show itself and this can result in many problems. These are dealt with under Male and Female Sexual Systems (pp. 87–95).

Careful **nutrition** is vital during pregnancy and the growing period; if anything it is more vital at those times than in ordinary adulthood. A fresh, balanced, natural diet is the optimum, free from over-processing and from artificial additives. Home preparation from fresh ingredients is the best way to secure this. If organic sources are possible, then that is best.

THE OLD DOG/CAT

The ageing have their own particular problems, as do the youngsters. In this section I shall draw attention to these and refer to the text in other parts of this book for detail. Old age should not be considered a disease, the aged should be allowed to spend the evening of their lives healthily, if possible, and to die healthy and in dignity when the end of their earthly journey is reached.

Leg Problems: All **arthritic** and **rheumatic** complaints become magnified in the old animal but usually respond in a very dramatic way to correct homoeopathic prescribing and natural dietary management. The pain of **Hip Dysplasia** can be helped greatly by *Colocynth* along with other rheumatic/arthritic remedies described on p. 104 et seq. **CDRM** and general leg weakness are discussed on p. 100 and on p. 114.

Growths: Are more prevalent on older animals, especially dogs, and some can respond well (see p. 124).

The **Heart, Kidneys** and **Eyes** are also prone to greater problems in the older patient but the treatment for these is adequately covered in the relevant pages of this book, that is, pp. 98, 85 and 60 respectively.

Ageing in general can produce loss of hair (consider *Thallium*), deafness, loss of elasticity in the tissue in general and progressive weakness; consider *Agnus castus*, *Argent. nit.*, *Causticum*, *Conium*, *Lycopodium*, *Silica* and *Thiosinaminum*. Sometimes these processes can be slowed and complaints arising from such processes can be improved markedly. A good natural diet is vital.

Ageing dogs often are **restless** at night causing themselves and their owners great disturbance. *Coffea* or *Arsen. alb.* have proved useful in these circumstances.

Collapsed animals and **terminal** patients can also be helped by appropriate remedies, apart from helping the heart as necessary. Reference to pages 121 and 128 can give encouraging results. In terminal disease the eventual duty of euthanasia must not be shirked if circumstances demand, but it is surprising how often a natural and dignified end can occur if proper homoeopathy is practised, especially if a natural diet and natural medicine have been used throughout the animal's life.

One should not start out by believing that an old dog or cat can be rejuvenated, ageing processes reversed or terminal illness suddenly evaporated by the use of homoeopathy in the aged but its results should not be ignored. One should not deprive the aged pet of such beneficial, gentle and easy remedies as can apply to their special case, for these remedies can, if not add on years (and in some cases they do appear to do this) to the animal's life, most certainly improve the quality of life left to such dignified creatures. The aged must not be deprived of their dignity by relentless illness.

CHAPTER 14

Homoeopathy in the Prevention of Disease

A system of medicine which does not recognise the need for prevention of disease is a non-starter to the sound minded observer. Homoeopathy not only recognises it but it has an unrivalled ability, in certain fields, to prevent disease.

Canine Parvovirus held the unenviable position of being the most notorious dog disease at the time of the first edition but is being very well contained by conventional vaccination in recent times. However, breakdowns are not unknown and younger puppies can present a real problem. The *nosode* prepared from Parvovirus, however, can give us very real protection in any age of dog (see Chapter 11 on Specific Disease, Appendix 11 Nosodes and page 154).

Nosodes can be prepared from **Distemper, Leptospirosis, Hepatitis, Kennel Cough,* Feline Enteritis, FeLV, FIP, FIV, FIA, Cat 'flu, Chlamydia, Staphylococcal infections, Canine Herpes virus, Myxomatosis** of rabbits **Paramyxovirus** of pigeons and any other infective agent one wishes. A regime of dosing over the first six months of life is usually required with subsequent six monthly doses to reinforce protection. Not only do these *nosodes* appear very effectively to prevent a disease, without side effects or allergy, they can also greatly assist in the curing of the disease should it already have occurred. Professional advice on this subject should be sought since this form of homoeopathy must be considered as a type of vaccination although the author does not use this term for it in his work. Your veterinary

---

* IJVH Vol. 2 p. 45 Kennel cough (plus corrections and clarification in Vol 2 No 2 p 57)

surgeon is best able to put these regimes into the correct context of your home and your pet and he can also obtain new *nosodes* made up to suit your circumstances. As a general rule a preventive course of *nosode* for any given disease would consist of the following regime: A dose twice daily for a few days followed by monthly doses for up to six months of age, followed by six monthly reinforcement doses. These *nosodes* can also be used in the situation where a previous illness caused by one or other of these infectious agents has left a permanent mark on the patient's health (see pages 41 and 125 and Chapters 8/13).

Prevention of other foreseeable problems can be effected by the use of appropriate remedies. For example impending **parturition**: *Caulophyllum*, as has been seen in Chapters 8–13, has its sphere of action primarily in this field and can be used to extraordinary effect both in the treatment and prevention of parturient problems. **Surgical shock** or ill effects can be prevented by the use of *Arnica, Calc. fl.* or *Staphisagria* (see Chapters 8–13). **Anaesthesia** hangover can be prevented by the use of the appropriate remedy e.g. *Chlorpromazine, Halothane, Opium* etc. **Eclampsia** can be prevented by the use of *Calc. phos.* **Dental calculus** tendency can be lessened by regular dosing with *Fragaria*. All acute prescribing with homoeopathy is an attempt at 'preventive' medicine, since the correct remedy should forestall any tendency of the disease to go 'chronic'. It also in many cases prevents death or euthanasia or even surgery where conventional medicine is often unable to avert these dire consequences. Who can question the unrivalled power of *Arnica* and *Aconite* to prevent many of the ill effects of injury and associated **shock**? **Blood loss** into the tissue is lessened and, as a result of this alone, further local tissue damage is prevented. **Rickets** and other disorders of bone growth can be prevented by *Calc. carb., Calc. phos.* and *Mag. phos.* Serious **scarring** after injury can be lessened or prevented by the use of *Thuja* and *Silica* by mouth and by *Calendula* topically. The use of *Mercurial* remedies in the treatment of **eye ulcers** can totally prevent further damage to the cornea. The ability to treat the unborn **in utero** (an interpretation of the term Eugenics) presents infinite possibilities for the prevention of disease, since disease in the pregnant dam can create miasmatic influences in the foetus. Emotional, dietary and infective conditions can influence the foetus seriously as can such problems as vaccinosis and other chronic diseases (see also pp. 42, 93 and 153). All can be treated during gestation to try to prevent ill effects on the foetus.

The veterinary surgeon taking up homoeopathy will be delighted with the chance that this form of medicine gives him to control, mitigate or totally prevent many problems and conditions which hitherto had eluded his attempts at control, the items listed here being but an introduction to the world of homoeopathic preventive medicine.

Trial work to prove the efficiency of nosodes in the prevention of Parvovirus, Distemper, Hepatitis, Leptospirosis or Feline Enteritis has not yet been performed (see Appendix 6 p. 208). Since there are no field outbreaks of these diseases in which to conduct clinical trials to test the efficacy of the nosodes, laboratory animal experimentation would be necessary to prove efficacy; a step the author is not prepared to take. Kennel Cough trials have, however, given dramatic results and much work has been reported on diseases in farm animals and in catteries (influenza). These would seem to show that the nosode system is effective in principle but, until a sufficient number of complete and fully-controlled clinical trials have been performed, owners must accept that the efficacy of these preventive remedies is unproven. Despite this cautionary remark, a great deal of anecdotal evidence has been built up over the years and users of the nosodes report no problems and great confidence; their animals having withstood outbreaks of disease in their locality. No breakdowns have come to the author's notice in animals treated with a correct and full regime of ethically-prepared nosodes. The weight of this anecdotal evidence is overwhelming, and will, I am sure, be supported by statistical data in due course.

CHAPTER 15

The Relationship of Homoeopathy to Conventional Medicine and Diagnosis

It is often remarked that it is not possible to use homoeopathic remedies either after conventional therapy or in conjunction with conventional therapy. As intimated in Chapter 2, I strongly believe that both these extreme statements are false although the ideal may be valid. Firstly, I have successfully treated with homoeopathy a great many cases which have received conventional therapy immediately beforehand. Secondly, I do, on rare occasions (as stated in Chapter 2), utilise conventional therapy alongside homoeopathy to palliate disease in the terminally ill. Thirdly, when patients are already on conventional therapy they cannot always be abruptly taken off when homoeopathy is commenced; the conventional drugs must often be 'tailed off'. Homoeopathy has often been shown to work even during the tailing-off period. Also, there are those cases where one fails homoeopathically for one of many reasons (again see Chapter 2) and one cannot then deny the patient conventional therapy if there is a chance that it will do good. There is no room for dogma in medicine if one is not to be guilty of neglect of one's duties to patients (see Hahnemann's quote p. 11). Other therapies and diagnostic techniques can be brought in where considered helpful e.g. Acupuncture,*

* Acupuncture and homoeopathy should be compatible but I am suspicious that they may not always be satisfactorily used simultaneously since they both attempt to shift energy patterns in the body. Their simultaneous use may invoke the problems associated with overprescribing (pp. 47/48, 53, 156) and consequently confuse or weaken the vital force. I now use one or other alone at any one time unless I can establish an integrated programme, as is possible in some cases. Use of one at a palliative level and the other at deep level may be effective simultaneously. It is a fact that the Chinese support acupuncture with herbs (among other things) and homoeopathy can fulfil this supportive role if used in a properly integrated fashion. Many homoeopathic

Anthroposophy, Bach Flower remedies, Biochemic Tissue Salts, Chiropractic, EAV, AK, Iridology, Radiaesthesia, Magnetic, Vibratory, Laser, Ultrasonic and Electrical therapies, Herbalism, Essential Oils (Aromatherapy), Osteopathy, etc.[†] All may have a place from time to time and the byword of the ethical physician, whether human or veterinary, must be open-mindedness.

In more detail, then, under which circumstances might conventional therapy argue with Homoeopathy? Firstly in the case of Corticosteroid or, less seriously, Antihistamine therapy, it is believed there is a very real chance that homoeopathic treatment can be blocked. Prior to a homoeopathic remedy being prescribed on the similia principle, in cases where such drugs have been used, one can use the 'potentised' form of whatever conventional agent is involved in order to speed its elimination from the system (p. 43). *Nux vomica, Sulphur* and *Thuja* are also excellent remedies for 'clearing' the system of previous treatments. Heavy long term corticosteroid therapy can often prove nearly impossible to clear, leading to total failure of natural therapy. Secondly, over-prescribing of conventional drugs and over-long treatments can seriously 'muddle' the case, confuse the symptomatology and lower the 'vital force' of the patient. (Similar comments can be made about gross over-prescribing of homoeopathic remedies too (see Chapter 6 pp. 47/48, 53, 155).) *Nux vomica* or *Sulphur* may be used to 'clear' the case when such muddles have occurred but not with guaranteed success.

There are, in contrast, many cases where homoeopathy can actually undo the harm done by some conventional therapies. The harmful effects of radiotherapy and cytotoxic therapy can be helped by similium prescribing and by potencies of the relevant agents. Even *X-ray* exists as a homoeopathic remedy. Vaccines may cause problems

remedies match the 'meridians' of Traditional Chinese Medicine and can also be appraised in terms of Yin and Yang. Remedies can also be found to correspond to the 'pernicious influence' pathways and synergise with TCM in that way (lecture by the author to IVAS Conference, Minneapolis, 1993)

[†] I am certain that these therapies are complementary to each other. Where Homoeopathy fails another may prove useful. Radionics may possibly be subject to similar constraints as those postulated for Acupuncture in footnote * above. The list of therapies has been expanded from the 1st Edition as a result of the author's widening use of different therapies and cooperation with practitioners of such therapies.

and here one might use *Thuja* (but see p. 149), possibly followed by the appropriate *nosode* or potentised *adjuvant*. Over-digitalised patients may be helped by *Nitric acid* or *Cinchona*. Patients over treated herbally can be helped by *Nux vomica*. *Aloe* has a reputation for helping those patients who have received too much antibiotic. The potentised forms of *Corcicosteroids, Hormones, Antibiotics*, NSAID's and *Anaesthetics* can all be used in an attempt to reverse their respective ill effects. When more research is conducted many more such practices may well emerge as being beneficial (pp. 41/42).

As stated in Chapter 2, adherence to veterinary homoeopathy does not mean the end of such commonsense practices as fluid and electrolyte therapy, nutritional therapy, surgery, nursing, management and, for veterinary surgeons, correct communication with the pet owner. Nor does it mean the end of such necessary diagnostic procedures as auscultation, thermometry, urinology, haematology, X-radiology, bacteriology, virology, parasitology, ophthalmoscopy, ulrasonography etc.; although these procedures may nowadays often be over-used at the expense of clinical observation and acumen. The homoeopath cannot hold himself above these things if he is properly to serve his patient. He may find himself relying less and less for diagnosis on such tests, as he progresses however (for it is true in general terms that modern methods and customs tend to rely on them too greatly, slowly losing respect for clinical instinct). Veterinary training can place too great an emphasis on 'science' and too little on the important philosophical and practical attributes of the real clinician, but there still must be a place for such tests and they should not be totally shunned.*

The modern homoeopath should set about reaping the benefit of the wealth of scientific lore which has accumulated since Hahnemann's day, putting it in its correct perspective, and combine all this with what he knows of the nature of disease, the nature of 'cure' (in the real meaning of the word) and the nature of medicine, gleaned from his

---

* On the matter of diagnosis itself, the conventional diagnostic approach, with its intended end product of a specific name for any disease in question, is not such a relevant concept in Homoeopathy. I refer you to pp. 13, 19, 37, 115, 213/214 also to the Organon of Hahnemann, Paras. 5–18 and 81 in which he expands upon this point very lucidly. However, the findings of such tests should take their place among the list of 'symptoms' characterising a case.

study of Hahnemann's work and from his own open-minded and philosophical approach to life. Surely, in doing so, he will establish that real ethic of veterinary medicine which can be directly lifted from Hahnemann's view of the physician's ethic so often quoted in this book (p. 11).

Vaccinosis: The varied problems arising from vaccination are worth singling out for special attention at this point. I have alluded to this problem elsewhere (p. 149, Glossary and IJVH Vol. 2 No. 1 p. 45 and Vol. 2 No. 2 p. 57 (corrections and clarifications)). It is not a well-documented fact that vaccination could be an erroneous strategy but evidence is building up, for those who wish to see, that all is not right with vaccination theory.* If such shreds of evidence (albeit often subjective) are not committed to paper for fear of ridicule then the problem will never be addressed by the scientific community and many valid observations from other veterinarians may never see the light of day (for it is very often the case that observations which appear to fly in the face of current wisdom are misjudged by the observer and not recorded until such time as others record similar observations).

Occult vaccinosis is a term coined by the author to describe disease arising remotely from vaccination and difficult to attribute with certainty to it. In individuals with a weak immune system it may conceivably be behind many cases of eczema, arthritis, epilepsy, allergy, autoimmune diseases, pancreatic insufficiency, immune deficient syndromes, feline gingivitis, miliary eczema and even Key Gaskell syndrome, vaccine being sufficient stimulus to throw the immune system off balance. Warts may also be predisposed by vaccination. A high proportion of cases of these diseases have been observed to commence within three months after a vaccination event, commonly after the first course or even after a double booster course, which

---

* The author is not alone in his fears with regard to vaccinosis. Other authors have also referred to their fears and there are references to it, in homoeopathic literature, going back a long way, even to Hahnemann, Organon, footnote to para. 56. It is probably to Dr James Compton Burnett that the credit must go for a full appraisal of the phenomenon (Vaccinosis and Homoeoprophylaxis). He refers to a diseased state of the constitution which has been engendered by vaccination. (An excellent treatise occurs in Homoeopathic Drug Pictures by M.L. Tyler, who reports Burnett's work very clearly.) Even Jenner's early work has had doubt shed upon its veracity and the accuracy of data reported therein has been thrown into question.

is often given by veterinarians after a period of neglect of annual boosters. This latter is a very sad occurrence since there is so little scientific support for the practice of annual boosting in the first place. Furthermore many cases of such conditions have appeared to improve with homoeopathic treatment only to relapse after booster vaccination, giving a clue to vaccine's possible involvement in their aetiology. The author considers German Shepherds to be particularly susceptible to 'occult vaccinosis', possibly as a result of a relative and general immune frailty, compared to other breeds.

Overt vaccinosis: Blue Eye in Afghan hounds with older, poorly-refined hepatitis vaccine, brain damage in humans following whooping cough vaccine, anaphyllaxis, frank illness following vaccination, lymphadenopathy, tonsillitis, etc. have all been witnessed as direct and obvious sequelae to vaccination.

Irish setters are particularly prone, in my opinion, to a tonsillitis following from vaccination. Haematological changes may also occur. Cavalier King Charles Spaniels may be similarly susceptible but more consistently also react locally to the injection. I have no theory as to why there should be these particular breed susceptibilities but the pattern has emerged over the years.

I believe that it is beyond doubt that there is a problem. What is open to doubt, however, is just how big that problem is and this presents a huge open field for research. It is going to be very difficult for anyone to acquire watertight proof of such a problem, mostly owing to the inbuilt time lapse involved. What is important however is that we must not hastily discard the benefits of vaccination without a great deal of humane research into its effects and possibilities for refinement or without the establishment of proper alternative regimes, since no-one wishes to see the horrendous effects of the virus killer diseases reemerge.

Alternatives. The *nosodes* present a very promising alternative for the protection of our animals against infectious disease. Work is being carried out on Distemper *nosode* and results of a trial on Kennel Cough (albeit on too small a scale) have been published (in IJVH Vol. 2 No. 1 p. 45 and clarifications Vol. 2 No. 2 p. 57). In practical terms the *nosodes* have been shown to prevent the development of disease in in-contact animals in catteries with cat 'flu, in kennel cough outbreaks and in many farm disease situations. There was also a trial showing the benefits of this method in bovine mastitis published in IJVH Vol. 1 No. 1 p. 15, 1986 (see also Chapter 14 and Appendix 6 and 11).

The danger of airing a discussion such as this is that it runs the risk of creating anti-vaccination fear and prejudice of an unenlightened nature, leading to total lack of protection of animals against such killer diseases as Distemper, Parvovirus, Panleucopaenia, etc. This is clearly not the author's intention. The purpose of the discussion is to stimulate forward-looking and to throw light on possible lines of therapy for some of the chronic diseases mentioned.*

Treatment of vaccinosis: Such remedies as *Pulsatilla*, *Lachesis*, *Silica*, *Sulphur* and *Thuja* are known to be able to help the body to throw off the problem of vaccinosis. More specifically, the various *nosodes* and potentised *adjuvants* can be considered in an attempt to 'antidote' the effects of the particular fraction of the vaccine thought to be causing the problem. There are even antibiotics in some vaccines and these can cause reactions. Do not forget the similium or the appropriate constitutional remedy, because this is arguably the only homoeopathic route to a complete cure.

---

* The author has even noted a possible connection between vaccination and the onset of cardiomyopathy and of heart valve disease (in which latter there is also considered by some researchers to be an immune component).

CHAPTER 16

Selected Case Histories

These cases are chosen to demonstrate the method of selection of remedies and to give some indication of how the possible sequelae manifest themselves (see Chapter 6). Potencies are given here for the first time in the book. This section is not advising in this matter but merely reporting potencies used. The cases are grouped according to the level of prescribing chosen (see Chapter 5).

TREATMENT OF THE ROOT CAUSE/ UNDERLYING PATHOLOGY

1   **An eighteen month old female cat admitted in emergency after a road traffic accident.** This cat was collapsed, breathing badly, pale and seemingly paraplegic. It appeared that the pelvis was broken and perhaps other injuries too but close examination would have been too distressing for the patient at the time. The case appeared to be bad enough for euthanasia but the patient was given *Arnica 30* at 15 minute intervals. By lunchtime that day the cat was making very good efforts to walk. 24 hours later an X-ray showed a dislocated hip and multiple fractures of the pelvis. The patient was now quite strong enough for anaesthesia so the hip as replaced and cage rest over the next 3 weeks effected an apparent total recovery. *Arnica 30* was given sporadically over the first three days.

2   **A two year old female cat brought in after a possible road traffic injury.** The cat was barely conscious, lying on its side and bringing up

copious bright frothy blood from its lungs. *Arnica 30* was administered every 5 minutes for half an hour then, since the cat brightened up enormously, only every two hours. This was an unexpected positive outcome but can probably be explained in retrospect by the theory that the haemorrhage was due to severe bruising of the lungs rather than gross tissue damage. Of course, it should be noted here that the availability of homoeopathic therapy bought this patient time which otherwise may not have been given in a case with such a grave condition.

3   **A six year old male Jack Russell Terrier had been lame for almost a month in mid February**. The stifle joint in that leg had been found to be very loose, painful and noisy on movement. Rest had been advised for three weeks with stifle surgery at the end of that period if no improvement was observed. The pain was causing a great deal of depression in the patient and he was not able to move about much at all, even though the leg was always carried. Homoeopathic treatment was sought and instituted in mid March. A mixture of *Rhus tox.*, *Ruta grav.* and *Arnica* all in **30c** potency was given twice daily for 10 days. Although the presenting symptom would have seemed to suit *Bryonia* better, the possible pathology to muscles, ligaments and periosteum, along with the resultant bruising and fear of being touched, were all considered more important. Great improvement was noted after the 10 days, not only in the ability to use the leg but in the personality and health of the patient. Again after three weeks more improvement was noted. After a further month, improvement had reached a plateau and *Rhus*, *Ruta* and *Arnica* in the **200c** followed. Improvement again took place and surgery was averted.

4   **A four year old Chihuahua female was brought in having previously had a stifle operation with prosthesis**. Ever since this the stifle had not been used properly and there had been a pink coloured discharge from the area periodically. It was decided to treat according to the pathology of a chronic suppuration rather than the historical line of treating for trauma to the joint. *Silica 30* was used three times daily for one month. Improvement was noted after two weeks and the discharge lessened. After several months the discharge was noted to be sporadic but the

leg was back in use. *Silica* was used from time to time thereafter and a constant but gradual improvement in the use of the leg was noted throughout. The discharge ceased. It was assumed that the homoeopathic medicine had helped to eliminate the chronic infection.

MENTAL LEVEL OF PRESCRIBING

1   **An eight year old male Golden Cocker Spaniel was showing successive signs of disease since February**: Itchy skin, epistaxis, pain in the hindquarters and, by October, abject lethargy, overweight, skin troubles and lack of 'sparkle'. He had been treated down the months conventionally and all but 'cured' of each of his symptoms. Thyroid treatment had come closest to producing a lasting effect. Homoeopathic treatment was started in December of that same year on the basis that in the previous December his lifelong companion a 10 year old bitch Cocker had been put down and that he was still, in the owner's opinion, grieving for her. *Ignatia 30c* was used twice daily for just one week. After one month a distinct improvement in all aspects of his health was noted followed by a relapse, but to acceptable levels. The improvement in his sense of well being was especially reported. A further three day course of *Ignatia 30c* was prescribed. This again elicited a marked response to even better levels but again something of a relapse soon after. After two more episodes of improvement and relapse the owner reported a failure to obtain improvement overall. *Ignatia 200c* was prescribed once daily for three days, repeat as necessary. No more *Ignatia* was required. An uneventful recovery was reported. Most of all the owner was pleased to report the return of the patient's '*joie de vivre*'.

2   **A year old Golden Retriever bitch was involved in a car accident as an occupant of one of the cars.** This was on the way to the owner's office. Ever since that day (several months previously) the dog had dreaded going to the office and sat under the desk and shivered all day long. Leaving the dog at home all day was unacceptable so homoeopathic treatment was sought. One dose of *Aconite 1M* was given followed by a week's course of *Gelsemium 30c* one daily. Here the

historical aspects of the case were used as well as the presenting mental symptoms. An immediate improvement was reported and no further treatment was necessary.

3 **An eight year old Collie cross male castrate was presented with chronic diarrhoea signs**, a quick and nervy nature, a stary coat and a fear of noises. No straining or pain was noted with the watery diarrhoea. *Merc. sol. 30* was given twice daily for three days. The diarrhoea stopped but the nerviness became worse. The dog was afraid to leave the house. Since the chronic diarrhoea had stopped coincidental with the treatment, *Merc. sol. 200* was chosen in order to obtain a deeper effect, despite the fact that the newly clarified mental symptoms did not quite fit. No result was obtained. *Argent nit. 30c* was then prescribed twice daily and an immediate improvement was noted. No further diarrhoea occurred and the nerviness was no longer a problem. This demonstrates the need to return to first principles in prescribing following a relative failure of the first prescription. It is especially important to take into account any new symptoms or changes following the initial prescription.

4 **A six and a half year old Gordon Setter male was presented in November with epileptiform fits which had started in May.** Clinically he was a nervy dog with a 'nervy' heart. Upon close questioning it was elicited that the fits usually occurred if one of the family was away. *Ignatia 30* was prescribed twice daily for one week. Two months later no fits had occurred but the patient was biting his feet. He had always done this apparently before he ever showed signs of fits, although the history taking had failed to discover this historic symptom. This was interpreted as a recapitulation phenomenon and *Ignatia 200c* was prescribed to be followed, if effective, by *10M* to achieve a deep and enduring effect. The condition resolved uneventfully.

5 *A note of caution* would not be amiss at this juncture. **A Cocker Spaniel came in very recently with epileptiform seizures** which started when the family moved house. The dog had been a rescue case and it was assumed the house move had brought about resurgence of the mental stresses previously undergone. Epileptiform fits, which were

refractory to conventional therapy, were occurring every 10 days. *Ignatia 30* was prescribed but was followed by a severe aggravation. The dose rate chosen of one twice daily for four days was obviously too great and two days later he suddenly went down with nine fits in one day! This was stopped by heavy conventional therapy by a neighbouring colleague and a cautious return to homoeopathy will be instituted soon, when it is certain that this effect has worn off. If fits become less frequent now it is certain *Ignatia* is the correct remedy.*

TREATING AT THE PRESENTING SYMPTOM LEVEL

1   **An eight year old male neutered cat had received a bite on his right fore foot**. Infection had travelled up the leg to the elbow. The animal was very ill and running a temperature. There was much pain and sensitivity. *Hepar sulph. 30c* four times daily was prescribed and the report two days later was of a very fit cat with a slightly sore leg. All symptoms were gone at the end of the week. No antibiotic was necessary.

2   **Near the end of May a 2 year old female Bulldog** came in by referral, the owner not wanting the bitch to undergo an ovarohysterectomy for the **pyometra** from which she was suffering. Polydypsia, pyrexia, lymph nodes swollen and inappetance along with a pinkish purulent vaginal discharge served to confirm the diagnosis. *Sabina 12c* and *Sepia 30* were given both twice daily. By the end of May the owner was happy that a complete recovery had occurred. Treatment was stopped. A check-up at the end of June confirmed the owner's opinion. Ovaro-hysterectomy had been avoided.

3   **A four year old neutered female cat was presented, after months of eye treatment, with a keratocoele on the right eye accompanied by corneal oedema, vascularisation and pigmentation.** She was sightless in that eye at the time. *Merc. sol. 30c* was prescribed since there was little photophobia or apparent pain. Intermittent treatment with the

---

* Since recording this case it was found that there followed a nine-week fit free period. A higher potency of *Ignatia* was then selected and given in single sporadic doses as necessary.

remedy produced a marked but gradual response for two months, after which time only a tiny white mark on the cornea remained. The order of cure was firstly the keratocoele, secondly the pink colouration to that area, thirdly the vascularisation which receded towards the limbus and fourthly the pigmentation which appeared to peel off, presumably as the cornea desquamated. This case illustrates the remarkable healing power of the eye under homoeopathic guidance. The very dramatic signs of chronic damage to the eye would normally lead one to expect the worst. However, once a healing spiral had been initiated, the signs resolved one by one to almost total resolution. Sight was also restored, since there had apparently been no damage to the lens or retina.

4 A three year old Wolfhound bitch was referred with a 'congenital' heart problem. She displayed very poor exercise tolerance, cyanosis, dyspnoea and inappetance. She had been badly deteriorating for the previous three months but had never been really fit as a youngster. The heart sounds were rounded and diffuse and the rhythm was erratic with tachycardia. *Digitalis, Crataegus* and *Viscum album* mixed liquid remedy was given. A check one week later revealed that the tongue was properly pink, exercise tolerance was good, there was more crispness to the heart sounds but the rhythm had not returned to normal. *Spartium 3c* pillules and *Convallaria* Ø tincture were given, but a check after a week showed no further improvement in the heart or the patient.

Spartium and *Dig./Crat./Visc.* were then adopted on alternate days for one month, then less frequently. The patient seemed to do very well and the heart sounds were good. She was not seen again until eight months later when she returned with rapid breathing, but she was still alert. Upon examination she was found to be suffering from constipation after eating a bone. *Alumina 30c* four times daily and increased frequency of *Dig./Crat./Visc.* tincture was prescribed to minimise the stress on the heart. Two days later all was well again. Six months after this a regime was adopted of one drop of *Dig./Crat./Visc.* mixture three times weekly with no *Spartium*. Six months later again, she suffered from a brownish discharge after an abnormal normal 'heat'. She was grumpy which she had never been before. She was given *Sepia 30c* and responded in two days. Her heart coped very well throughout life and she lived to a natural 'old age'.

5 **An eighteen month old West Highland White bitch came in with Keratitis Sicca (Dry Eye).** Four months previously the other eye had been affected, treated unsuccessfully with conventional therapy for one month and then had been submitted for surgery (parotid duct transplant). This had ameliorated the condition but the initial damage to the cornea remained. When the second eye became affected it was Easter time and no referral for surgery was possible. Homoeopathic treatment and artificial tears were immediately instituted while surgery was being booked. *Zincum met. 30c* twice daily was the treatment and artificial tears as necessary. It soon became obvious that artificial tears were needed less and less often until eventually the impending operation was cancelled and the artificial tears stopped. There was no damage to the eye and it was still completely healthy, without further treatment, one year later.

6 **A three year old British Blue neutered male was brought in suffering from an intractable rodent ulcer** which had worsened despite conventional therapy for more than 6 months. The face was seriously disfigured. *Con. mac.* and *Nitric acid* were prescribed, both in 30c. Within a week the paws broke out in lesions which discharged white creamy pus. His skin also broke out in lesions resembling miliary eczema. Both of these lesions had been displayed by this patient in the previous summer to his rodent ulcer appearing. This was assumed to be a *recapitulation* process and therefore an indication of a correct remedy. However, after an initial improvement in the ulcer for one month no more improvement seemed to occur. The treatment was changed to *Merc. sol. 30c* along with *Galium Ø* tincture and *Calendula* lotion on the ulcer. Foot aggravation and skin aggravations again occurred. *Nitric acid* and *Merc. sol.* were used on different occasions for a period of one year and finally the lesion on the face disappeared and the face remodelled so that it appeared normal. For the last six months of treatment one *Merc. sol. 200c* pillule per week or fortnight was prescribed depending upon response.

7 A queen whose milk would not dry up was given *Cyclamen 30c* by the owner, since this had previously been successfully prescribed for a similar condition in another queen. Since no response was shown quickly, a four times daily treatment was given for three days. The cat became ill, off her food, very slow and pyrexic. She was then brought in for veterinary attention and no mastitis or other disease could be found. The *Cyclamen* was stopped and the symptoms subsided almost immediately. This was a proving of some of the symptoms of *Cyclamen* which had been given too frequently and for too long and was the wrong remedy. *Urtica 1x* then dried up the milk.

8 A kennel of Shelties suffered an outbreak of diarrhoea and vomiting. The first puppy to contract the disease showed the symptoms of *Merc. sol.* (that is, wet mouth, thirst, yellow frothy vomit, painless diarrhoea, inappetance and smelly breath). It responded in a few hours to a **30c** potency. Successive members of the litter contracted similar symptoms and were given the same remedy by the owner and responded, except one. When the owner discussed this non-response it was found that there was clear mucoid vomit and tenesmus with the diarrhoea in the affected puppy. *Merc. cor. 30c* was given and the response was rapid. This illustrates the need for close observation of symptoms and concomitants and for willingness to change the remedy accordingly.

General Note. In a sensitive patient aggravations provings and recapitulations can occur very readily on what may appear to be a very low dose of remedy. Each patient is different, and treatment 'according to results' is the only way to take this into account. Rigid application of dosage regimes, without taking response into account, can create difficult problems.

TREATMENT OF HISTORICAL PROBLEMS

1 A 9 year old Rottweiler male was referred with a history of upper respiratory problems. There was noisy breathing, but no discharge, sneezing or other sign of disease. There was no history of tooth troubles and none could be found. The noisy breathing had started about 5 months previously. During the history-taking, previous medical history revealed an operation to the right stifle coincidentally about five months previously. It was this historical event which was selected as the crucial point for prescribing since it was considered feasible that his palate or pharynx could have undergone bruising during or after anaesthesia. He was still lame on the stifle so the same pathology could have been instrumental in both symptoms. *Rhus tox.*, *Ruta grav.* and *Arnica* (all in **30c**) were prescribed and within two weeks the breathing was fine and the leg much better. A slight relapse of both symptoms after three weeks demanded a further short burst of treatment and then only the leg had occasional relapses.

2 A working Collie was brought in because it had lost its sight. The owner related it to a minor head injury about a year previously. He claimed that the vision had gradually been lost ever since that event so that now the Collie's useful life as a cow dog was finished at the age of two years. The eyes appeared to be normal by ophthalmoscopy but the dog was referred to a specialist anyway. No abnormalities were found. On the strength of the owner's conviction, *Arnica 200c* was prescribed, one pillule weekly. After one month the dog was back in work and suffered no relapse. It was assumed, retrospectively, that there must have been some pressure on the optic nerves in the skull, possibly as a result of old haemorrhage, which was resolved by the *Arnica*.

CONSTITUTIONAL PRESCRIBING

1 A three year old Chihuahua bitch had been exhibiting erratic hormone cycles. When she was on heat it appeared thoroughly normal with normal bleeding. She had been mated three times but with no success. She was a timid creature with little thirst. *Pulsatilla 30c* was prescribed and a report eight months later stated that she had since brought up a litter of puppies.

2 A seven year old Chihuahua bitch was exhibiting a very dirty coat. The coat was greasy, smelly and sparse. This condition had been continuing unabated for three years. The dog had a sad demeanour. Since the patient actually sought out somewhere warm to lie, rather than be cool, *Psorinum 30c* was chosen rather than *Sulphur*. Within two weeks great improvement was seen in the coat and in the liveliness of the patient. After one month there was no more trouble.

3 A four year old domestic shorthair cat (female neuter) showed miliary-eczema-type lesions on her back, flanks and over her head. These would forms crusts and were accompanied by hair loss, extreme itchiness and irritability. The skin appeared otherwise unchanged. This particular cat was fearful of noises, was very independent, voluntarily spent most of her time indoors and was quick to anger. She also had a great liking for salty foods if offered. She was given a single dose of *Natrum mur. 30c* to which she responded rapidly, the skin signs disappearing over the following three weeks.

4 An eight year old female neuter domestic long hair cat was presented with a history of skin trouble, characterised by sores, scabs, hair loss, redness and heat. She was a great liker of cream and sweet biscuits. Her skin symptoms were generally worse in the heat of summer and she was not a cat to enjoy the warmth of the central heating boiler or the airing cupboard. It was considered that she required *Sulphur 200c* and after three doses at weekly intervals, her skin started to improve dramatically. After one month, a single dose of *Sulphur 1M* appeared to resolve the case fully.

These cases are not reported with the intention of 'proving' that homoeopathy works but rather as illustrations of the way in which it can be used. Many of the possible sequelae to treatment occurred in these few cases. Consistent reports from clients whose animals are on the correct remedy nearly always include a reference to the improved overall health and well-being of the patient, and very often include reference to the increased amount of sleep in the first twenty-four hours. This latter finding may stem from a possible lack of rest in disease and the extra sleep being needed to catch up on that deficit.

CHAPTER 17

A Short Materia Medica
of some Key Substances

This chapter inevitably cannot contain a note on every homoeopathic medicine nor even a full coverage of the major ones, or it would be a book in itself. The text is therefore confined to the main points of some major remedies and of a few lesser ones, in order to help in the use of the book (particularly Chapter 8) as it guides you to basic remedy selection. The bibliography (Appendix 5) will help in choosing further reading.

Aconitum napellus (Aconite). One of the great fever remedies. Associated with fear nearly always, its symptoms are sudden in onset. Eyes are red and inflamed with watery discharge. There is usually photophobia. Ear pinna may become red, hot and swollen. There may be nosebleeds of bright red blood usually with a sneeze. There may be signs of soreness of the throat. Vomiting with thirst is seen and a painful abdomen. Urine may be red and hot. There is a hoarse cough with tachycardia and a full bounding pulse. *Aconite* is famous for its effect in cases of shock. Symptoms may be brought on by or aggravated by cold dry winds, but its indications are any sudden and dramatic disturbance of the patient's equilibrium. For a fuller dissertation on the veterinary application of *Aconitum*, refer to BHJ Vol. 82 pp. 97–105 April 1993.

Actaea racemosa (Cimicifuga racemosa). With its affinity for the musculoskeletal system, nervous system and female sexual systems this remedy is used mostly in these contexts. Restlessness of the limbs, stiffness and spasm in neck and back regions, chorea and jerking, pain in lumbar and sacral regions are all seen. Ovarian and uterine symptoms are often associated with the locomotor problems. Symptoms are usually worse in the morning and better for warmth.

Allium cepa. Frequently turned to in cases of coryza where there is a profuse watery discharge, bland from the eyes but acrid from the nose. There is often photophobia. There can be a hoarse cough, and symptoms are usually worse in the evening or in a warm room and better for open air or cold room.

Aloe socotrina. The diarrhoea symptoms often govern the choice of this remedy. There is distended abdomen, the stool may be passed involuntarily with much flatus. The stools are often mucoid and the anus sore. The remedy is also useful to re-establish health after long, heavily-treated illness, where symptoms are confused, especially after prolonged use of antibiotics.

Alumina. Debilitated old patients showing weak muscles and constipation characterise the remedy's main prescribing points. Mucous membranes and skin tend to be dry and inflamed. One can therefore see conjunctivitis, otitis externa and dry, hard stools passed with much straining. Sometimes there is absence of desire to pass the stool because of the general paretic state. Nails are often brittle. Symptoms are worse in the morning and in a warm room, better for open air and in the evening.

Ammonium carbonicum. Indicated where there is wheezing and laboured respiration, typically in overweight patients with a weak heart and probably showing a harsh cough. The nose may be stopped up at night and there may also be nosebleeds. There may also be urinary incontinence at night. Symptoms are worse in evenings and in the middle of the night, worse for wet and cold, better for dry weather.

Antimonium tartaricum. A remedy characterised by a loose rattling, unproductive cough, such as is often heard in cats. Respiration can be very difficult with much gasping, often associated with marked cyanosis. There is usually thirst for little and often. Symptoms are worse in the evening, lying down, and in cold damp weather or a warm room.

Apis mellifica. This remedy is of great use in conditions characterised by shiny oedematous swellings which 'pit' on pressure. There is usually a great desire for open air, particularly if there is respiratory involvement (e.g. pulmonary oedema). *Apis* is suited to conjunctivitis with chemosis (in which the conjunctiva 'bubbles' out), acute or chronic pulmonary oedema, swollen shiny joints, and also in cases of nephritis with urine retention. It has a diuretic action too. It is particularly of use in cases of vulval injury, where oedema can prevent urination, such as may occur after a traumatic birth process. Symptoms are worse for heat or touch, better for open air and cold bathing.

Argentum nitricum. Purulent ophthalmia with abundant discharge, corneal ulceration and corneal opacity are all symptoms of this remedy. Trembling nervousness, particularly if it leads to stomach disorders or diarrhoea, also responds well. Symptoms are worse for warmth and at night, better for fresh air and cold.

Arnica montana. This is homoeopathy's great *injury* remedy and should be used in all cases of injury and surgical interference, especially dental extraction. Bruising and ecchymoses characterise its symptoms, also fear of being touched. It is often forgotten that it has powerful antiseptic properties too. It can be used internally or topically as a lotion or ointment. It is also of use to help symptoms of over-exertion.

Arsenicum album. Anxiety or restlessness are often present where this remedy is indicated. Discharges from eyes or nose are watery and acrid causing ulceration in those regions. The mouth is usually dry and the patient is usually thirsty. Dramatic vomiting and diarrhoea, often simultaneously, indicate its use if concomitant signs agree. The patient may have wheezing respiration, and allergic asthmatic conditions can respond well. The skin can be dry, scaly and scurfy. Skin and respiratory signs alternate. An important constitutional remedy. Symptoms are worse for cold and wet, better for warmth.

Belladonna. This is one of the great fever remedies, conditions requiring its use usually being of *violent* nature and sudden onset. Heat, redness, pain and swelling characterise its symptoms. It is one of the many remedies of use in convulsions. Pupils are usually dilated, so its use in *Key Gaskell Syndrome* in cats is well known but it is only one of many in this condition also. Acute ear inflammations where there is heat, pain and swelling respond well. The mouth is usually dry and there is a great thirst. Symptoms are worse for noise, touch, or jarring motion and better for quiet, dark, rest and slight warmth.

Bellis perennis. As with *Arnica* it is useful for injury but more especially deep muscular bruising or pelvic injury. Think of it therefore post partum, for instance, and after deep orthopaedic surgery. Where there is stumbling and weakness in late pregnancy it is also indicated.

Bryonia alba. This remedy shows both diarrhoea and constipation symptoms, the latter usually in chronic conditions. The mouth is often dry and there is a great thirst. It is of great help in many cases of rheumatism or arthritis where symptoms agree (see page 104). Part of its picture can be respiratory signs with a hoarse, hacking cough. Mastitis will respond if modalities are correct. All symptoms are *markedly worse for movement* and better for rest (p. 104).

Calcarea carbonica. A constitutional remedy of major importance, classically of use in overweight, slightly sluggish patients usually displaying skeletal disorders or delayed or abnormal dentition. Lameness symptoms include an unwillingness to stretch out the affected limb when lying. Eye symptoms include pupil dilation, blocked lachrymal ducts or even cataract. Chronic catarrh can occur. There is usually an increased appetite which may be depraved. Lymph nodes in the throat are often enlarged and there may, in addition to bone growth abnormalities in the young, be umbilical herniation. The skin has an unhealthy appearance and a tendency to warts. Symptoms are usually worse for exertion, cold and wet; better for dry weather.

Calcarea fluorica. Is especially useful where hard swellings feature among the symptoms. Glandular swellings and mammary growths are an example. Bony malnutrition of puppies can be helped and it has a reputation for helping control adhesions after abdominal surgery. Symptoms are worse for rest and damp, better for exercise and warmth.

Calcarea phosphorica. This remedy is similar in action to *Calcarea carbonica* but suits better the leaner patient. Bony puppies, appearing out of proportion, showing a depraved appetite, delayed dentition, epiphyseal malformation and arthritic changes resulting from this, all indicate this remedy. Patients are often more active than those suiting *Calc. carb.* Symptoms are worse for cold and damp, and better for warm dry conditions (p. 104).

Calcarea sulphurica. Slow healing, discharging, purulent lesions respond well to this remedy. Discharges are usually yellow. It can help chronic catarrh, cystic growths and thick, yellow discharges. In contrast to *Silica* it is most effective when discharges have found an outlet.

Calendula officinalis. Is chiefly used topically, as a lotion or ointment, applied to wounds and abrasions. It promotes rapid healing and controls sepsis, having a great value on open wounds and ulcers. Its popular and effective use in this way should not lead one to forget that it can be taken internally to aid wound healing and help ward off infection of wounds. Dilute mother tincture (ø) to make a lotion.

Cantharis vesicatora. This is an irritant poison with a predilection for the urogenital system and skin. Hence homoeopathically used classically in cases of cystitis where painful straining is a feature, with blood in the urine. Urine is usually passed in tiny amounts very frequently, some unproductive efforts also being made. Skin lesions are vesicular rashes. Burns and scalds respond to this remedy. Symptoms are worse for touch, better for rubbing.

Caulophyllum. This remedy is primarily used in all conditions *relating to parturition*; before, during and after. It controls and aids parturient relaxation of the tissues, uterine contractions, expulsion of the foetus, expulsion of the foetal membranes and, finally, involution of the womb. This is if it is given as a prophylactic measure. When this has not been done, it is still of great use at any stage and can even help to resolve post parturient metritis. This remedy is also associated with pains in the small joints especially if these are during or after pregnancy (p. 104) (see also Veterinary Record*).

Causticum. A remedy whose prime action is on the neuromuscular system† and skin. Warts which are rough, and flat respond well. Rheumatism better for warmth and generalised stiffness also call for *Causticum.* Chronic cystitis and intertrigo also may respond. Symptoms are worse in cold dry conditions, better in warm damp conditions. A constitutional remedy (p. 94).

Chamomilla. Primarily known for its action on *teething* problems it can bring relief to a great many health problems arising at the nursing stage and after, in young animals. Conditions which arise at this time may be skin problems, epilepsy, diarrhoea, colic, swelling of the lymph nodes and abdominal tympany. In nearly all cases there are signs of an irritable response to pain or interference. Nursing problems in the mother (e.g. painful mammae) and even false pregnancy may respond.

Chelidonium majus. A liver remedy of major importance, its symptoms are those of obstructive jaundice, congested liver, diarrhoea alternating with colic, stool yellow or clay-coloured depending upon whether there is obstruction of the bile system or not. Symptoms are usually worse for movement and touch and early mornings, better after food. The patient, when ill, tends to prefer the chill taken off drinking water.

Cinchona officinalis. This is Hahnemann's historic *Peruvian bark.* Periodic fevers, sweats, cold skin and great debility are the main sphere for *Cinchona.* The pulse is usually thready and weak, haemorrhages, when present, are usually dark clots. There is sensitivity to touch. It should always be considered in dehydrated patients after illness. Symptoms are usually worse for touch, draughts and after food, better for warmth and open air.

---

* Veterinary Record March 1984 Vol. 114 p. 216.   † Paretic tendency.

Cistus canadensis. Hard glandular swellings typify this remedy, especially those of throat and neck and the mammae. The mouth is usually cold and smelly with swollen gums. When growths ulcerate and when the patient feels the cold badly, *Cistus* could be of help. Ears often show a watery purulent discharge.

Cocculus. Inability to open the mouth or swallow, with drooling and vomiting in some cases, indicate *Cocculus*. It acts on the central nervous system and is therefore an '*epileptic*' remedy. Symptoms are always worse for prolonged movement so it is one of the *travel sickness* remedies.

Coffea cruda. Acts upon the nervous system to produce restlessness, agitation and sleeplessness, particularly in the small hours. Hyper-sensitivity of skin, intolerance of pain and discomfort after food with bloated abdomen are classical *Coffea* symptoms. Symptoms are worse for noise and better for warmth.

Colchicum autumnale. With *Colchicum* there is coldness and pros-tration and usually a gassy, distended abdomen. The patient is unwilling to allow the legs to be stretched out. There is thirst and craving, but offerings of food are then refused. This often fits the picture of the hunting cat with a gassy tummy, inappetance, inactivity and coldness. It is also of use in some forms of arthritis, usually when joints are red, hot and swollen. Symptoms are invariably worse for movement (p. 94).

Colocynthis. A remedy for *spasmodic colic* where, as with *Colchicum* but more markedly, the legs are hunched up, compressing the abdomen. There may be a tight distension of the abdomen and there is usually a flatulent diarrhoea which produces temporary relief. There is usually much mental agitation. The patient often grinds teeth and is worse for noise. Hip pain may respond, making this a useful remedy in cases of painful hip dysplasia.

Conium maculatum. The remedy is characterised by weakness and trembling, particularly in the aged and particularly starting at the hind limbs. Ageing symptoms of the eyes and limbs especially can be helped, as are many tumours especially those of the lymph glands and mammae. Chronic ulceration may also be associated. With eye symptoms pain is uppermost. It is the first choice remedy for old dogs with weak hindquarters. Symptoms are worse when lying down or rising and from exertion but are better for motion.

Crataegus. A heart tonic remedy, helping irregularities of rhythm, weakness from chronic heart disease, oedema of dependent parts or generalised oedema (dropsy), dyspnoea on least exertion, dilated heart, weak heart sounds and valvular murmurs. Usually given as ø.

Digitalis. As with *Crataegus* this is a heart remedy, for use when pulse is weak, irregular and slow, but quickened by least effort, when the heart is weak and dilated, when dropsy occurs and when there is a tendency to fibrillation. The tongue may become blue. The patient may even be helped when actual heart failure has occurred.

Drosera rotundifolia. Coughing with retching or vomiting is a good indication for this remedy. Spasmodic dry coughing attacks following closely upon each other, along with changes in the voice, are characteristic. It appears as if something were caught in the throat. Symptoms are worse for lying down, for warmth, after midnight and for swallowing or excitement.

Euphrasia. This remedy is mainly of use in conjunctivitis where there is photophobia, catarrhal corrosive discharge, sticky mucus on the cornea, and frequent blinking. Symptoms are worse for warm winds, evening, light and better in darkness. Use in the form of eye drops as well as internally. Dilute mother tincture (ø) to make eye drops.

Gelsemium sempervirens. Mentally this remedy is useful for anticipatory fear, show fright, fear of thunder, some forms of epilepsy and in excitable male dogs. Fear and nervousness can lead to urination and can root the patient to the spot. There is usually some weakness and trembling in the limbs. Luxating patella is an interesting indication for its use, in which it often produces marked amelioration of symptoms. It has been used successfully to treat nystagmus following cat 'flu.

Symptoms are worse for damp, impending storm, excitement, better for open air and continued activity.

Graphites. A constitutional remedy, it is indicated in the fat, lazy, smelly-skinned dog which enjoys the fireside. The skin is usually dry and itchy, hair falls out and ears and eyes have a watery, purulent discharge. The skin in the folds of the limbs may crack and discharge a clear, sticky fluid. Symptoms are worse for warmth and at night.

Hamamelis virginica. Extravasation of blood, ecchymoses, passive venous haemorrhage which fails to clot (dark, seeping haemorrhage), weakness from loss of blood and pain in large open wounds or post-operative pain can all be greatly helped by *Hamamelis*. Aids resorption of blood clots.

Hepar sulphuris. A major remedy for use in cases of *suppuration*. Typically lesions are very sensitive to touch. It should be used to prevent suppuration when specific injury has occurred (e.g. cat bite) and should also be used if signs of suppuration have developed. It aids resorption of pus (e.g. hypopion) and treats cellulitis. Symptoms are worse for touch and cold, better for warmth.

Hypericum perforatum. Reduces pain in open, lacerated wounds and in closed injuries where tissues are rich in nerve endings (e.g. crushed toes or tail). Post operative pain and spinal injury may be greatly helped and it should be used, along with *Ledum*, to prevent *tetanus* developing from puncture wounds. The remedy is often used as a lotion, combined with *Calendula*, to treat painful grazes or open wounds. Symptoms are worse for cold and touch.

Ignatia. *Ignatia* should always be considered where there is evidence of insecurity or agitation arising from abandonment, *bereavement* or loneliness. This can be triggered by loss of a human or animal companion. Hysteria, self mutilation, skin disease, epilepsy and general fading can all result from the above emotions and close history taking can often reveal their involvement, even at some defined stage in the past. It has also been successfully used in weaning problems in mother or offspring.

Ipecacuanha. Vomiting repeatedly, associated with respiratory embarrassment call for this remedy. Attacks can lead to collapse. Nose bleed of bright red blood and similar haemorrhages from the womb, blood in the milk of suckling mothers and post-operative vomiting are all good indications for its use. Symptoms are worse as lying down and show a periodicity.

Kali bichromicum. Is characterised by *yellow ropy* discharges. It acts mainly upon the membranes of the eyes, gastro-intestinal tract and respiratory system. The eyes show swelling of the lids, the characteristic discharge and even corneal ulceration. Pain is not usually a prominent feature in the latter. Chronic catarrh again shows characteristic discharge, rawness of nares and obstructed nose. If there is a cough it is productive, again with characteristic expectoration. Urine is similarly affected. Vomiting will usually produce bright yellow water and the stools are brown and frothy. Symptoms are worse in the morning and in hot weather but better from local heat.

Kali carbonicum. Great weakness and intolerance of cold weather with irritability and hypersensitivity are properties of this remedy. Sac-like swellings appear in upper eyelids and eyelids stick together in the morning. The nose becomes blocked in a warm room. Nasal discharge is yellow and thick, but not viscid, nostrils are made sore and ulcerate. In the female weakness and debility after parturition is seen, in the male weakness after coition. A wheezing cough with or without hydrothorax can be seen. Symptoms are worse for cold weather, and in the small hours; better for warm weather and for movement.

Kali chloricum. Essentially its action lies in destructive kidney disorders, especially chronic nephritis with putrid breath, acrid saliva, ulcerated mouth. If there is diarrhoea it is greenish. Urine albumen and phosphates are high and there is often blood.

Ledum palustre. Think of this remedy in conjunction with puncture wounds (also *Hypericum*). It has a strong *antitetanus* reputation and also aids wound healing. Symptoms are worse at night and for heat, better for cold.

Lilium tigrinum. This is one of the great female constitutional remedies, suiting a patient which tends to rush about and flit from one activity to another. The patient is usually depressed and fidgety. There is congestion of pelvic organs with offensive bloody discharge from the womb while moving, ceases when still. There is often an urgent desire to defaecate, with an increased thirst. It is one of the remedies used in pyometra in bitches (p. 92).

Lycopodium clavatum. This remedy exerts most of its effect on the digestive organs, liver, kidneys and respiratory system. The patient dislikes being left alone and appears apprehensive. The nose can be blocked and there may be blisters on the tongue. Eating a little food tends to satisfy the very marked appetite. The belly is usually bloated. The stool appears small and hard and is expelled only with difficulty, accompanied by ineffectual straining. Urination is also a slow process and urine has a red sediment. There is often an irritating cough. Symptoms are worse for heat generally and better for cold. An important constitutional remedy.

Mercurius corrosivus. Aptly named, this constitutional remedy acts on corrosive destructive processes. The ears discharge greenish pus, with ulcers in the ear canal. The eyes show acrid tears, often with corneal ulceration and intense photophobia. The eyelids are reddened with excoriation. Mouth ulcers appear and the breath is foul with profuse, acrid saliva. The alimentary system is similarly affected, great thirst being present with much vomiting of clear mucoid fluid. Diarrhoea is painful, producing much tenesmus. The kidneys undergo similar corrosive changes leading to haematuria and albuminuria. There is also tenesmus on urinating. Purulent wet eczema with extreme pain often responds to this remedy. Symptoms are worse evening and night, better resting.

Mercurius solubilis. A very similar remedy to the above, but showing less dramatic symptoms. There is usually no photophobia, chronic vascularised eye ulcers respond well, vomit is usually yellow and there is no tenesmus with the diarrhoea. High potency suppresses suppuration.

Natrum carbonicum. A *thunder* remedy. It can be of help in heat exhaustion, milk-induced diarrhoea, chronic catarrh, especially if odorous, and patients subject to easy spraining of joints. Symptoms are worse for summer heat, thunder storms, draughts; better for movement.

Natrum muriaticum. This is the homoeopathic medicine made from common salt. Despite its lowly and commonplace origins it is a powerful and far-reaching constitutional remedy. Mentally, the animal can be fearful and seek solace in its own company. There is an aversion to direct sunlight and a fear of loud noises (e.g. a vacuum cleaner). The animal usually likes salt, can be thirsty and chilly and often displays problems of fluid or electrolyte imbalance. The coat is greasy. The female may be aggressively unwilling to mate (see p. 91).

Natrum sulphuricum. Should be remembered in cases of *head injury*, possibly resulting in brain damage. Also in cases of meningitis. There is usually photophobia. The abdomen is flatulent and diarrhoea (especially in the morning) is involuntarily passed with flatus. Symptoms are worse for damp weather, better for dry weather.

Nitric acid. A notable wart remedy (for those which bleed easily) it also acts strongly on mucocutaneous junctions. Lesions which are around this region respond well (e.g. rodent ulcer). Any lesion which bleeds freely should lead one to consider this remedy and extreme pain is often a symptom. Symptoms are worse for hot weather and at night time.

Nux vomica. Primarily used in the digestive sphere, its greatest reputation is in helping disturbances following *overeating of unsuitable foods*. Faeces is usually hard but diarrhoea can follow overeating. There is abdominal discomfort, flatulence, irritability and sensitivity to noise. It is also used in cases of umbilical herniation in young animals, and can often help the extreme muscle spasm with difficult urination after *disc prolapse*. It is one of homoeopathy's 'clearing' remedies, and a great constitutional remedy. Symptoms are generally worse for noise, worse in the morning and better after rest or for damp weather.

Petroleum. This remedy is very useful in preventing *travel sickness*. Skin symptoms which also call for it are dryness, cracks, redness, rawness, easy bleeding. There can be dry lesions around eyes and ears. Symptoms are worse in damp weather and from travelling, better for warm air and dry weather.

Phosphoric acid. One of several remedies of use in debility, especially if diarrhoea is present. There is usually apathy, dehydration and loss of condition. There can be an association with grieving. Diarrhoea is usually yellow and of a painless nature. It can help regulate bone growth and tends to suit the youngster who has been overtaxed or over exercised during the growing period. Symptoms are worse for exertion, better when warm.

Phosphorus. A very 'sudden' remedy. The patient is sensitive to loud and sudden noise (e.g. thunder storms, fireworks etc.). Degenerative processes and bone destruction respond to *Phosphorus*. Food is suddenly vomited back when it has been warmed in the stomach. Gums can be ulcerated and bloody. Hepatitis, jaundice, pancreatic disorders and nephritis come into its sphere. Urine may be bloody. A very painful cough is also a symptom affecting the whole body. Wounds which perpetually bleed can be helped. The patient is usually in poor body condition. *Phosphorus* is an important constitutional remedy. Symptoms are worse for touch, exertion, evening and during thunder storms; better for cold and sleep.

Phytolacca. Glandular swellings are its greatest field of action, usually associated with debility and restlessness. Lymph nodes and mammary gland swellings are red, hard and sensitive. Throat involvement is common, with difficult swallowing and red discolouration. There are also shifting rheumatic symptoms and a tendency to boils. Symptoms are worse for exposure to damp, cold weather, motion and at night; better for warmth, dryness and rest.

Picrid acid. Neurasthenia, notably in oversexed male dogs, characterises this remedy. Also weakness associated with prostate problems in old dogs. Young dogs who are overstimulated sexually can reach a state of near paralysis with foaming mouth. Extruded penis is also a sign. Symptoms are worse for exertion and in wet or hot weather, better for cold.

Platina metallicum. One of the predominantly female constitutional remedies. An aloof-seeming patient usually over-hungry with irregular and abnormal hormone cycles is typical. Usually the abnormality tends to nymphomania rather than diminution of sexual behaviour (see p. 91).

Podophyllum. Primarily a diarrhoea remedy, it is characterised by colicky pain, sometimes vomiting of bile and gushing offensive stool, which contains mucus and is usually painless. There is often a greenish colour to the watery faeces. There can also be a concomitant prolapsing of the rectum. Symptoms are worse in early morning and in hot weather.

Psorinum. Besides *Sulphur* this is the best known '*mange*' remedy. It is the *nosode* of the human scabies vesicle. Its symptoms are a smelly dirty skin and coat, scurfiness and chilliness in a patient which craves heat. It is a constitutional remedy. Symptoms are worse for changing weather, cold and hot sunshine; better for warmth.

Pulsatilla nigricans. One of homoeopathy's great 'female' constitutional remedies (see p. 91), suiting best the patient of shy, yielding disposition. Disorders of the female hormone system respond well when the type fits. Discharges, whether from nose, eyes, vulva, etc., are creamy and tend to a greeny/yellow colour. Another pattern which responds well is that of symptoms which *come and go*, e.g. appetite, diarrhoea, itchy eyes, shifting lameness, etc. There is usually little thirst. The patient is cheerful but easily dispirited. Symptoms are worse for heat, towards evening; better open air, motion, cool.

Pyrogenium. Valuable in toxaemic febrile conditions, especially where there is a weak pulse. Think of it in puerperal fevers and where discharges are putrid. Think also of *Echinacea* in this connection.

Rhus toxicodendron. Is the most famous of the *rheumatic* remedies. The skin and musculoskeletal system are its main spheres. Small red papules in the skin, and sometimes vesicles, are typical skin lesions, with much scratching. Cellulitis may occur. In all cases of damage to muscles think of *Rhus* and the symptoms of arthritis/rheumatism which respond are those which are worse after rest, particularly if this follows strenuous exertion. The symptoms improve with limbering up, only worsening on excessive exertion. Classically the worst pains and stiffness are seen as the animal rises from its bed (p. 104).

Ruta graveolens. A powerful remedy in cases of sprain or dislocation. If there is any damage to fibrous structures such as tendons, ligaments or periosteum turn to *Ruta*. Symptoms, as with *Rhus*, are worse after rest.

Sabadilla. This remedy helps sneezing coryza with red sore eyes. The throat can be affected, causing frequent swallowing movements. The patient is sensitive to cold. Symptoms are worse for cold and better for warmth.

Sabal serrulata. Its greatest reputation is in the treatment of prostatic disease. Loss of sexual power and general evidence of irritability of the urogenital system indicates its use. In the female, underdeveloped mammae may be helped.

Sanicula. Indicated when discharges have an offensive fishy odour. It has proved of use in recurring anal gland problems where this has been used as a pointer. Painful constipation, where desire only occurs after great quantities accumulate, expelled with great difficulty. The stool often recedes and crumbles. 'Fishy' vaginal discharges are a further symptom. Travel sickness cases can also be helped, in patients displaying a fear of downward motion. The symptom picture bears remarkable similarity to that of *Silica*.

Sarsaparilla. Primarily a urinary remedy, being particularly effective in cases of urethral obstruction. Sabulous plugs or calculi can both respond. There is usually tenesmus, pain and blood. This remedy has its most fruitful application in cases of *feline urological syndrome* when it fits the above picture.

Sepia. A famous 'female' constitutional remedy, notable for its effect on the 'darker' mental side of female hormonal aberration. False pregnancy bitches with unpredictable bad temper typify it. Pelvic organs are usually slack with a tendency to prolapse. Membranes may be slightly yellowed and the patient is sensitive to cold (see p. 91). General indifference is its great hallmark. Symptoms are worse for cold air and before a thunder storm; better for exercise, warmth and after sleep.

Silica. This constitutional remedy fits the shy, chilly patient who is reluctant to enter the consulting room. Chronic inflammatory conditions such as sinuses and granulomata respond well. If the cause should be a *foreign body*, then so much stronger the indication. It is surprising how often a foreign body such as a grass seed, splinter, thistle or thorn (or even bone fragment from an injury) can create a low grade inflammatory response in the body, which fails to eject it. If abscessation and discharge occur then the lesions frequently heal and open again and again. Use *Silica* in such situations and be prepared for a long term treatment (as long as three weeks in some cases).

Spongia. The coughing patient with little exercise tolerance, congested lungs and resting for long periods in sternal recumbency is a good subject for *Spongia*. The cough is usually better after eating.

Staphisagria. This remedy is associated with the mental state of resentment which is difficult to define in animals. We can often guess at this state from the history or from the demeanour. It is also of use in post-operative complaints, especially if near orifices and in problems in maiden bitches after their first mating.

Stramonium. This is a *convulsion* remedy primarily. Some cases of epilepsy respond. Pupils are dilated. The patient prefers light to dark. Graceful rhythmic rather than jerky choreic movements of limbs are characteristic. Symptoms are worse alone, in the dark; better in company, in the light.

Sulphur. This is the most famous '*mange*' remedy. Constitutionally the typical patient is dry, dirty coated, smelly, overweight and stubborn. It dislikes heat and chooses, if possible, to lie on a cold floor. However, it is arguably homoeopathy's largest remedy, about which a book could be written in its own right. The symptomatology is so large that it is able to mimic and overlap with a great many other homoeopathic medicines. The skin is typically red over the whole patient. Mucocutaneous junctions are nearly invariably reddened. Difficult respiration can occur, with a desire for open air. If concomitant symptoms agree, both diarrhoea and constipation can respond. This remedy is one of the homoeopath's weapons for 'clearing' the system of overtreatment or poisoning. Symptoms are worse for heat and at rest.

Symphytum. Its common name is 'knitbone' and this is its main action – promoting effective healing of fractures. It should be used in all such cases (along with *Arnica*) to ensure adequate callus formation and optimum resolution. It is effective in combating the effects of peri orbital, and eye injury (sclera) too. If you have no *Arnica* in your first aid kit, *Symphytum* can assume its mantle for all injuries.

Thuja occidentalis. A wart remedy of primary importance when warts are pedunculated. Anal adenomata may respond. When adverse reaction to vaccination has occurred *Thuja* can offer almost immediate relief in some cases. It is a constitutional remedy, the patient being typically chilly, with symptoms worse at night and in cold, damp air.

Urtica urens. *Urticarial* reaction in the skin responds well to *Urtica*, where acute irritation, small red weals and great agitation occur. Burns and scalds respond well (see *Cantharis*). Low potency suppresses *milk* in engorged mammae and high potency stimulates the flow. Agalactia may respond to treatment. Urinary suppression also indicates this remedy. Symptoms are not helped by cold water (cf. *Apis*) in fact the opposite is the case.

Veratrum album. Cases of *dysentery*, where the patient is cold, cyanotic and collapsed, indicate this remedy. The pulse is usually rapid and weak and the coldness very marked. The remedy helps to control dehydration and is one of the remedies useful in cases of coprophagy.

Viscum album. Lowered blood pressure with a slow pulse, respiratory difficulty, hypertrophic heart with valvular incompetence are characteristic. It is useful in the treatment of some *cancers*. Symptoms are worse in winter and for movement and the patient prefers sternal recumbency.

Zincum metallicum. A *convulsion* remedy where, in between fits, there is great depression. The patient is sensitive to noise but lethargic. The eyes roll and there can be conjunctivitis, especially in the inner canthus. '*Dry Eye*' can respond to this treatment. Colic occurs after eating. Symptoms are worse for touch and after food.

Glossary of terms met in this book and in Homoeopathic Literature in general

ACUTE DISEASE: Is one which is of rapid onset and short duration. It implies nothing of its severity. The outcome is death or recovery.

ADJUVANT: Material added to a conventional killed vaccine to enhance local reaction, with the intention of bettering resulting immunity.

AGGRAVATION: Worsening of symptoms associated with the administration of a correct remedy at an incorrect potency.

ALLOPATHY: System of medicine utilising agents to treat disease which are totally unrelated to the disease in their action.

ANTIBIOTIC: An antimicrobial therapeutic agent originally synthesised by living organisms (e.g. fungi). Now many are artificially synthesised.

ANTIOPATHY: System of medicine utilising agents to treat disease which are opposite to the disease in their action.

BLEPHAROSPASM: Spasm of the eyelids.

c: See Centesimal.

CENTESIMAL: Scale of dilution of a remedy, each stage being one in one hundred. Denoted by c.

CHEMOTHERAPEUTIC: A chemical agent used in conventional medicine to combat bacterial or protozoal infection e.g. Antibiotic, Sulphadimidine.

CHRONIC DISEASE: Is one which is of long standing and well established, there is no period of resolution.

COMPLEX REMEDY: A remedy of several constituents combined. Often different potencies of the same homoeopathic medicine or synergistic remedies combined.

COMPOUND REMEDY: A remedy made up of several or many different individual homoeopathic medicines. A system common in France and Germany.

CONCOMITANT SYMPTOM: Is one which accompanies the presenting symptom and is a useful aid to prescribing homoeopathically.

CONSTITUTIONAL REMEDY: Is one which takes the entire make up of the patient into account, rather than presenting symptoms and concomitants alone. The 'picture' includes all local and general symptoms, behaviour demeanour, likes, dislikes, physical appearance, mental symptoms, etc. The nature of the body's programmed response to disease is its constitution.

CORTICOSTEROID: A steroidal agent produced by the Adrenal Cortex or a synthesised analogue of this. Anti-inflammatory and highly suppressive in action (Steroid q.v.). Also called Cortisone.

CURE: The total elimination of disease and restoration of health.

d: See Decimal.

DECIMAL: Scale of dilution of a remedy, each stage being one in ten. Denoted by **d** or x.

DISEASE: Dynamic disturbance of the harmony existing between the 'Vital Force' in a body and the material body itself. Literally Dis-Ease.

ENDEMIC: Describes a disease (usually transmissible) which exists among a certain human population and usually reaches a balance with that population.

ENZOOTIC: As above but applies to animals.

EPIDEMIC:	Describes a disease (usually transmissible) which is not in balance with a human population and is spreading.
EPIZOOTIC:	As above but applies to animals.
EPISTAXIS:	Nose bleed.
EUGENICS:	In the context of this book, the word is taken to describe treatment of the unborn *in utero* as an attempt to eliminate disease acquired in utero as a result of maternal ill-health or miasmatic influence.
EUTHANASIA:	Humane killing of a patient, in order to avert suffering from terminal illness.
GENERALS:	Symptoms applying to the whole body.
HETEROPATHY:	See Allopathy.
HOMOEOPATHY:	Treatment of disease with a substance which has the power to reproduce, in a healthy body, symptoms similar to those displayed by the patient.
HOMOEOSTASIS:	The maintenance of equilibrium within the body with regard to all metabolites, body temperature, etc.
HYPER-:	Prefix denoting excess.
HYPO-:	Prefix denoting insufficiency.
IMMUNITY:	The ability to resist infection usually by means of circulating or tissue antibodies but can have a wider meaning, applying to the entire mechanism whereby homoeostasis is maintained and imbalance is resisted.
INTUSSUSCEPTION:	Telescoping of the bowel.
ISOPATHY:	Treatment of disease by the identical agent of the disease. Here vaccination has similarities (see also *nosode*).
LESION:	Change produced by disease in tissue or organ.
MALIGNANCY:	See Neoplasia.

MATERIA MEDICA: Book of provings of remedies, listing their symptoms and possibly their clinical applications.

MIASM: Hahnemannian term for infective agent. Literally 'cloud' or 'taint'. No direct definition in modern medical terms exists. From μιασμα (Greek).

MODALITY: Modification of symptoms by such influences as temperature, time, motion, weather etc.

MOTHER TINCTURE: Undiluted alcoholic solution obtained from original plant material. The starting point for all potencies from soluble material (denoted by Ø).

NEOPLASIA: Literally 'New Growth'. Usually reserved for cancer (also malignancy).

NOSODE: Remedy prepared from infected tissue, disease discharges or 'causal' organisms (see Isopathy).

NYSTAGMUS: Rhythmic, jerky movements of eyes, usually laterally, usually involuntary.

OPISTHOTONUS: Describes the posture of an animal in extensor spasm, that is, head and neck back, legs outstretched, back hollowed.

OVAROHYSTERECTOMY: Surgical removal of ovaries and womb.

PALLIATIVE: Treatment aimed directly at reducing symptoms (antiopathy).

PARENTERAL ROUTE: Route of administration of a medicine other than via the alimentary canal (e.g. by injection).

PARTICULARS: Symptoms applying to individual organs, organ systems or parts of the body.

PATHOLOGY: The science which deals with the cause of and changes produced by disease – usually confined to demonstrable physical tissue changes.

PHOTOPHOBIA: Literally 'fear of light'. Describes the spasmodic blinking of animals when confronted with light to which they are over sensitive.

PLACEBO: Medicine given to humour, rather than cure, the

	patient. A psychologically induced cure may follow – 'the Placebo Effect'.
POLYCREST:	One of the deep acting consistently applicable remedies which have a wide action on all parts of the body. Constitutional remedies are polycrests.
POTENCY:	The dynamic principle of a remedy harnessed in the dilution/succussion process. Quantified by c or x (d) and the number of stages undergone.
POTENTISATION:	The above process (Trituration q.v.).
PROSTHESIS:	Surgical insertion of foreign material, usually to correct anatomical deficiency or injury.
PROVING:	The administration of a remedy to a body sufficient to cause symptoms noted in the materia medica. In modern language it is a poor translation of the German: *Prüfung* – a test.
PYREXIA:	Fever.
RECAPITULATION:	In the context of this book, the recurrence of past elements of a chronic disease (often seemingly unrelated to present symptoms) as a result of homoeopathic treatment. These past elements are usually symptoms previously suppressed by Antiopathy.
REGULATORY REMEDY:	In the context of this book, a remedy which has opposite actions at high and low potencies.
REPERTORY:	Book of symptoms with indicated remedies (a dictionary of symptoms).
SIMILIUM:	A remedy closely matching the symptoms exhibited by the patient, the ideal homoeopathic remedy.
STEROID:	Sterol-related substances having a basic chemical configuration based on Cyclopentophenanthrene which is an unsaturated hydrocarbon. Synthetic analogues also exist (see also Corticosteroid).
SUCCUSSION:	The agitation process applied to homoeopathic remedies at each stage of dilution during the potentisation process.

SUPPORTIVE THERAPY: Arguably part of nursing rather than medicine. Applies to fluid, electrolyte and nutritional supplementation given to a weak patient. Blood transfusions, artificial lungs, oxygen therapy, renal dialysis, etc. may also come under this heading.

SYMPTOM: The homoeopaths' view is that a symptom is the result of the patient's fight against the disease. The discernible properties of the disease process in the patient by which one decides upon a remedy.

TENESMUS: Straining e.g. at faeces or urine.

THERAPEUTIC: Remedial.

TRITURATION: Serial dilution of insoluble material with milk sugar, prior to subsequent liquid dilution as per potentisation (q.v.). It is usually necessary to attain a dilution of 10^{-6} (ie 3c) prior to beginning liquid dilutions.

VACCINATION: Administration of live attenuated or killed disease agent in order to protect a patient against that or similar specific disease (see also Isopathy).

VACCINOSIS: Disease resulting from vaccination.

VITAMIN: Derived from 'Vital Amine'. Essential ingredients of diet playing a part in cellular chemistry, structure of tissues, function of nerves, integrity of membranes and immune responses. Supplementation can be an essential part of medicine and, for therapeutic purposes, levels may far exceed recommended daily amounts (RDA).

x: See Decimal.

Remedy List

There follows a list of the common names of remedies (where these differ from the Latin names) with their Latin equivalents and common abbreviations.

Common Name	Latin Name	Abbreviation
Aconite	Aconitum napellus	Acon.
Acrid Lettuce	Lactuca virosa	Lact. v.
Aloe	Aloe socotrina	Aloe
Aluminium Oxide	Alumina	Alum.
American Arum	Caladium seguinum	Calad.
Ammonium Carbonate	Ammonium carbonicum	Ammon. carb.
Ant	Formica	Form.
Apomorphine	Apomorphia	Apomorph.
Arbor Vitae	Thuja occidentalis	Thuja
Argilla	Alumina	Alum.
Arsenic Trioxide	Arsenicum album	Arsen. alb.
Atropine	Atropinum	Atrop.
Balsam Apple	Momordica balsamina	Momord.
Baneberry	Actaea spicata	Actaea sp.
Barberry	Berberis vulgaris	Berb.
Bichromate of Potash	Kali bichromicum	Kali bich.
Bitter Cucumber	Colocynthis	Coloc.
Black Lead	Graphites	Graph.
Black Snakeroot	Cimicifuga (Actaea) racemosa	Cimic. rac.
Blood Root	Sanguinaria	Sanguin.
Bluebell	Agraphis nutans	Agraph.
Blue Cohosh	Caulophyllum	Cauloph.
Blue Flag	Iris versicolor	Iris

Borate of Sodium	Borax	Borax
Bounafa	Ferula glauca	Ferula
Bromide of Potash	Kali bromatum	Kali br.
Bryony	Bryonia alba	Bryon.
Bugle Weed	Lycopus virginicus	Lycopus
Buttercup	Ranunculus bulbosus	Ran. b.
Bushmaster (Surucucu)	Lachesis	Lach.
Calabar Bean	Physostigma	Physost.
Calcium Carbonate	Calcarea carbonica	Calc. carb.
Camphor	Camphora	Camph.
Carbonate of Barium	Baryta carbonica	Baryta carb.
Carbonate of Lime (see Calcium Carbonate)		
Carbonate of Potash	Kali carbonicum	Kali carb.
Caroba Tree	Jacaranda	Jacar.
Cat Thyme	Teucrium marum	Teuc. mar.
Cayenne Pepper	Capsicum	Caps.
Cereus (see Night Blooming)		
Cevadilla Seed	Sabadilla	Sabad.
Chamomile	Chamomilla	Cham.
Chaste Tree	Agnus castus	Agn.
Cherry Laurel	Laurocerasus	Lauroc.
Chick Pea	Lathyrus sativus	Lathyr.
Chlorate of Potash	Kali chloratum	Kali chlor.
Christmas Rose	Helleborus niger	Helleb.
Club Moss	Lycopodium clavatum	Lycop.
Cobalt	Cobaltum	Cob.
Cobra	Naja tripudians	Naja
Cockroach	Blatta americana	Blatta
Coffee	Coffea	Coff.
Comfrey	Symphytum	Symph.
Condor Plant	Condurango	Condur.
Copper	Cuprum metallicum	Cupr. met.
Coral Snake	Elaps corallinus	Elaps
Corn Smut	Ustilago maydis	Ustil.
Corrosive Sublimate	Mercurius corrosivus	Merc. cor.
Cotton	Gossypium	Gossyp.
Cowhage	Dolichos puriens	Dolich.
Crawfish	Astacus fluviatilis	Astac.
Creosote	Kreosotum	Kreos.
Croton Oil Seed	Croton tiglium	Croton tig.

Cuban Spider	Tarentula cubensis	Tarent. cub.
Culvers Root	Leptandra	Lept.
Cuttlefish Ink	Sepia	Sep.
Cyanide of Mercury	Mercurius cyanatus	Merc. cyan.
Daisy	Bellis perennis	Bell. per.
Damiana	Turnera	Turn.
Deadly Nightshade	Belladonna	Bell.
	(Atropa belladonna)	
Duck Weed	Lemna minor	Lemna
Dusty Miller	Cineraria	Ciner.
Elder	Sambucus niger	Samb.
Ergot (of Rye)	Secale cornutum	Secale (Sec.)
Eyebright	Euphrasia	Euphr.
Figwort	Scrophularia nodosa	Scroph.
Flea	Pulex irritans	Pulex
Flint	Silica (or Silicea)	Sil.
Fluorspar	Calcarea fluorica	Calc. fluor.
Fool's Parsley	Aethusa cynapium	Aeth.
Fowler's Solution	Kali arsenicum	Kali ars.
Foxglove	Digitalis purpurea	Digit.
Fringe Tree	Chionanthus	Chion.
Galipea cusparia bark	Angustera vera	Angust.
Glauber's Salt	Natrum sulphuricum	Nat. sulph.
Goa	Chrysarobinum	Chrysarob.
Goat's Rue	Galega officinalis	Galega
Gold	Aurum metallicum	Aurum
Golden Ragwort	Senecio aureus	Senec.
Golden Seal	Hydrastis	Hydr.
Goose Grass	Galium aparine	Galium ap.
Gravel Root (see Queen of the Meadow)		
Greater Celandine	Chelidonium majus	Chel.
Ground Holly	Chimaphila umbellata	Chimaph.
Gypsum	Calcarea sulphurica	Calc. sulph.
Hawthorn	Crataegus officinalis	Crat.
Hedge Hyssop	Gratiola	Grat.
Hemlock	Conium maculatum	Con. mac.

Henbane	Hyoscyamus	Hyosc.
High Cranberry	Viburnum opulis	Viburn. op.
Honey Bee	Apis mellifica	Apis mell.
Horse Chestnut	Aesculus hippocastanum	Aesc. h.
Hydrochloric Acid (see Muriatic Acid)		
Hydrofluoric Acid	Fluoricum acidum	Fluor. ac.
Indian Cockle	Cocculus	Cocc.
Indian Hemp	Apocynum cannabinum	Apoc.
Indian Tobacco	Lobelia inflata	Lob.
Indigo	Baptisia tinctoria	Bapt.
Iodide of Arsenic	Arsenicum iodatum	Arsen. iod.
Iodide of Lime	Calcarea iodata	Calc. iod.
Iodide of Potassium	Kali hydriodicum	Kali hydriod.
	(Kali iodatum)	(Kali iod.)
Iodine	Iodum	Iod.
Ipecac Root	Ipecacuanha	Ipecac.
Iron	Ferrum metallicum	Ferr. met.
Jaborandi	Pilocarpus microphyllus	Piloc.
Jack in the pulpit	Arum triphyllum	Arum triph.
Jambol Seed	Syzigium	Syzig.
Jelly Fish	Medusa	Med.
Jequirity	Arbrus precatorius	Arbrus
Jerusalem Oak	Chenopodium	Chenop.
	anthelminticum	
Knitbone (see Comfrey)		
Kombe Seed	Strophanthus	Stroph.
Lead	Plumbum metallicum	Plumb. met.
Leopard's Bane	Arnica montana	Arn.
Lily of the Valley	Convallaria majalis	Convall.
Lucerne	Alfalfa	Alf.
Lungwort	Sticta pulmonaria	Sticta
Male Fern	Filix mas	Filix. m.
Mandrake (see May Apple)		
Mare's Tail (see Scouring Rush)		
Marigold	Calendula officinalis	Calend.
Marjoram	Origanum	Orig.

Marking Nut	Anacardium orientale	Anac.
Marsh Tea	Ledum palustre	Ledum
Meadow Saffron	Colchicum autumnale	Colch.
Mercuric Sulphide	Cinnabaris	Cinnab.
Mercury (see Quicksilver)		
Mistletoe	Viscum album	Viscum
Monkshood (see Aconite)		
Night Blooming Cereus	Cactus grandiflorus	Cactus
Nitroglycerine	Glonoinium	Glon.
Nutmeg	Nux moschata	Nux m.
Onion (see Red Onion)		
Orange Spider	Theridion	Ther.
Pasque Flower	Pulsatilla nigricans	Puls.
Passion Flower	Passiflora	Pass.
Pennywort	Hydrocotyle	Hydrocot.
Peony	Paeonia	Paeon.
Peruvian Bark	Cinchona officinalis	China or Cinch.
Pheasant's Eye	Adonis vernalis	Adon.
Phosphate of Iron	Ferrum phosphoricum	Ferrum phos.
Phosphate of Lime	Calcarea phosphorica	Calc. phos.
Phosphate of Magnesium	Magnesia phosphorica	Mag. phos.
Phosphate of Potassium	Kali phosphoricum	Kali phos.
Picrate of Iron	Ferrum picricum	Ferrum pic.
Pine Tar	Pix Liquida	Pix liq.
Pink Root	Spigelia	Spig.
Pipsissewa (see Ground Holly)		
Plaster of Paris (see Gypsum)		
Poison Ivy	Rhus toxicodendron	Rhus tox.
Poison Nut	Nux vomica	Nux vom.
Poison Weed	Wyethia	Wyeth.
Poke Root	Phytolacca	Phyt.
Pomegranate	Granatum	Gran.
Poppy latex	Opium	Opium.
	(Papaver somniferum)	
Potash Alum	Alumen	Alumen
Potassium Hydrate	Causticum hahnemannii	Caust.
Primrose	Primula obconica	Prim. obc.
Prussic Acid	Hydrocyanic acid	Hydrocyan. ac.

Puffball	Bovista	Bov.
Purple Cone Flower	Echinacea (Rudbeckia)	Echin.
Purple Fish	Murex	Mur.
Quartz	Silica (Silicea)	Sil.
Quebrachio	Aspidosperma	Aspid.
Queen of the Meadow	Eupatorium purpureum	Eup. purp.
Quicksilver	Hydrargyrum	Hydrarg.
	Mercurius solubilis	Merc. sol.
Quinine Sulphate	Chininum sulphuricum	Chin. sulph.
Radish	Raphanus	Raph.
Ragworth (see Golden Ragwort)		
Rattlesnake	Crotalus horridus	Crotal. horr.
Rattlesnake Bean	Cedron	Cedr.
Red Onion	Allium cepa	All. cep. (Cepa)
Red Starfish	Asterias rubens	Aster.
Rock Rose	Cistus canadensis	Cistus
Rudbeckia (see Purple Cone Flower)		
Rue	Ruta graveolens	Ruta grav.
Saffron	Crocus sativa	Crocus
Sage	Salvia officinalis	Salvia
Sal Volatile	Ammonium carbonicum	Ammon. carb.
Salt	Natrum muriaticum	Nat. mur.
Savine	Sabina	Sab.
Saw Palmetto	Sabal serrulata	Sabal serr.
Scabies Nosode	Psorinum	Psor.
Scouring Rush	Equisetum	Equis.
Shepherd's Purse	Thlaspi bursa (pastoris)	Thlaspi
	(Capsella b.p.)	
Silico Fluoride of Calcium	Lapis albus	Lapis alb.
Silver Nitrate	Argentum nitricum	Argent. nit.
Skullcap	Scutellaria	Scut.
Smilax	Sarsaparilla	Sarsap.
Snakewort	Senega	Seneg.
Snow Rose	Rhododendron	Rhod.
(Helleborus is also sometimes referred to as Snow Rose)		
Sodium Biborate	Borax	Bor.
Southern Wood	Abrotanum	Abrot.
Sowbread	Cyclamen	Cycl.

Spanish Fly	Cantharis	Canth.
Spanish Spider	Tarentula hispania	Tarent. hisp.
Sponge	Spongia	Spong.
Spurge Olive	Mezereum	Mez.
	(Daphne mezereum)	
St Ignatius Bean	Ignatia	Ign.
St John's Wort	Hypericum perforatum	Hyper. (Hyp.)
St Mary's Thistle	Carduus marianus	Carduus mar.
Starfish	Asterias rubens	Aster.
Stargrass	Aletris farinosa	Aletr.
Star of Bethlehem	Ornithogallum	Ornith.
Stavesacre	Staphisagria	Staphis.
	(Staphysagria)	(Staphys.)
Stinging Nettle	Utrica urens	Urt.
Stone Root	Collinsonia canadensis	Collins.
Sulphate of Lime	Calcarea sulphurica	Calc. sulph.
Sulphate of Potassium	Kali sulphuricum	Kali sulph.
Sulphide of Antimony	Antimonium crudum	Ant. crud.
Sundew	Drosera rotundifolia	Dros.
Surucucu (Bushmaster)	Lachesis	Lach.
Tartar Emetic	Antimonium tartaricum	Ant. tart.
Thornapple	Stramonium	Stram.
	(Datura stramonium)	
Thoroughwort	Eupatorium perfoliatum	Eup. perf.
Tiger lily	Lilium tigrinum	Lil. tig.
Tin	Stannum metallicum	Stan. met.
Toadstool	Agaricus muscarius	Agar.
Tobacco	Tabacum	Tabac.
Ucuba	Myristica sebifera	Myr. seb.
Valerian	Valeriana officinalis	Val.
Vegetable Charcoal	Carbo vegetabilis	Carbo veg.
Verdigris	Cuprum aceticum	Cupr. ac.
Virgin's Bower	Clematis erecta	Clem.
Virgin Vine	Pareira brava	Par.
Water Hemlock	Cicuta virosa	Cic.
White Bryony (see Bryony)		
White Hellebore	Veratrum album	Verat. alb.

Wild Cherry	Prunus virginiana	Prunus v.
Wild Indigo (see Indigo)		
Wild Liquorice (see Smilax)		
Wild Strawberry	Fragaria	Frag.
Wild Yam	Dioscorea villosa	Diosc.
Witch Hazel	Hamamelis	Ham.
Wolfsbane (see Aconite)		
Woody Nightshade	Dulcamara	Dulc.
	(Solanum dulcamara)	
Wormseed	Cina	Cina
Yarrow	Millefolium	Millef.
	(Achillea millef.)	
Yellow Dock	Rumex crispus	Rumex
Yellow Jasmine	Gelsemium sempervirens	Gels.

APPENDIX 3

Common Potency Levels

United Kingdom

Decimal potencies are rarely used but these are the potencies in which they commonly appear in the UK when available:

1x, 3x, 6x, (12x) these are low potencies.

Centesimal potencies are much more common. The customary potencies available are:

3c, 6c, 12c, 30c, 200c, M and 10M
3c is low. 6c and 12c are transitional. 30c and 200c are high.

M and 10M refer to dilutions of 1/100, one thousand times and 1/100 ten thousand times respectively. These are very high potencies and more rarely used in veterinary work.

6c is the commonly obtainable potency.

If no suffix letter appears then assume c, that is *Sulphur* 6 is in fact *Sulphur* 6c.

Mother tincture is denoted by the Greek letter Ø (see p. 203). Several remedies will appear in the text, recommended as mother tinctures.

Trituration: (see p. 194) is used for insoluble material.

Europe

European countries use different potencies from the United Kingdom, as their commonly prescribed remedies.

Firstly, instead of x suffix they use **d** prefix to denote decimal potencies. So 6x will appear as **d6**.

Secondly their common potency levels are:

c4 c5 c7 c9 c15 c30 etc.

alternatively:–

4cH. **5cH**. **7cH**. **9cH**. **15cH**. **30cH**. etc. are more common in France. (cH = centesimal Hahnemannienne)

Failure to understand this can contribute to confusion when meeting European remedies on holiday, where homoeopathic remedies are more widely obtainable than in the United Kingdom, or should you have such remedies in the cupboard from previous imports.

Other systems: You may find LM potencies mentioned, or Korsakoff potencies. These are beyond the scope of this small book.

APPENDIX 4

Useful Addresses

British Association of Homoeopathic Veterinary Surgeons
Hon. Secretary, Alternative Veterinary Medicine Centre, Chinham House,
Stanford in the Vale, Nr Faringdon, Oxon. SN7 8NQ. 01367 710324 (office),
01367 718115 (recorded message), 01367 718243 (fax)

British Homoeopathic Association
27a Devonshire Street, London WIN IRJ. 0171 935 2163

British Homoeopathy Research Group
Secretary, 101 Harley Street, London WIN IDF

British Small Animal Veterinary Association
Kingsley House, Church Cove, Shurdington, Cheltenham, Glos. GL51 5TQ.
01242 862994

British Veterinary Association
7 Mansfield Street, London WIM OAT. 0171 636 6541

Faculty of Homoeopathy
2 Powys Place, Great Ormond Street, London WCIN 3HT. 0171 837 9469

Homoeopathic Trust
Hahnemann House, 2 Powys Place, Great Ormond Street, London
WCIN 3HT. 0171 837 9469

International Association for Veterinary Homoeopathy
UK contact via BAHVS (see above)

National Association of Homoeopathic Groups
Secretary, 11 Wingle Tye Road, Burgess Hill, West Sussex RHI5 9HR

Royal College of Veterinary Surgeons
Belgravia House, 64 Horseferry Road, London SWIP 2AF. 0171 222 2001

Bibliography

	Materia Medica with Repertory	Boericke
†	Introduction to Homoeopathic Medicine	H. Boyd
*	Veterinary Toxicology (Garner's)	Clarke and Clarke
*	Bovine Medicine, Blackwells Scientific Press (Andrews) (Chapter 59 on Homoeopathy and Acupuncture)	Christopher Day, MRCVS
*	Feeding Dogs the Natural Way (Chinham)	Christopher Day, MRCVS
*	The Homoeopathic Treatment of Beef and Dairy Cattle	Christopher Day, MRCVS
*	Homoeopathy, First Aid for Horses (Chinham)	Christopher Day, MRCVS
*	Homoeopathy, First Aid for Pets (Chinham)	Christopher Day, MRCVS
*	Natural Remedies for your Cat (Piccadilly)	Christopher Day, MRCVS
*	Natural Remedies (for Horses) (Threshold Guide)	Christopher Day, MRCVS
*	Textbook of Veterinary Alternative and Complementary Therapies, Mosby (Shoen and Wynn) (Chapter 26, Veterinary Homoeopathy)	Christopher Day, MRCVS
	Homoeopathy First Aid in Accidents and Ailments	D.M. Gibson
†	Organon of Medicine 5th and 6th Edition	Hahnemann. (Dudgeon and Boericke)
†	Organon of Medicine (New translation)	Hahnemann. (Künzli, Naude and Pendleton)
*	Homoeopathic First Aid Treatment for Pets (formerly Before the Vet Calls)	Francis Hunter, MRCVS

Repertory of the Homoeopathic Materia Medica with Word Index	Kent
† The Handbook of Homoeopathy	G. Koehler
* Cats: Homoeopathic Remedies	George Macleod, MRCVS
* Dogs: Homoeopathic Remedies	George Macleod, MRCVS
* Goats: Homoeopathic Remedies	George Macleod, MRCVS
* Homoeopathy for Pets	George Macleod, MRCVS
* Pigs: The Homoeopathic Approach to Treatment and Prevention of Disease	George Macleod, MRCVS
* The Treatment of Cattle by Homoeopathy	George Macleod, MRCVS
* The Treatment of Horses by Homoeopathy	George Macleod, MRCVS
* A Veterinary Materia Medica	George Macleod, MRCVS
* Natural Health for Dogs and Cats	Pitcairn and Pitcairn
Synthesis (Repertorium Homoeopathicum Syntheticum) (Homoeopathic Book Publishers)	Dr Frederick Schroyens
Homoeopathic Drug Pictures	M.L. Tyler
Concordant Materia Medica	Vermeulen
* Homoeopathic Medicine for Dogs (Translation)	H.G. Wolff

JOURNALS (see Appendix 6)

COURSES (see p. 29)

† Useful books on the principles of Homoeopathy in general
* Purely veterinary books

The others (unmarked) are of great use and relevance. Although purely human in content, much can be adapted for veterinary use.

APPENDIX 6

Research

This is a brief outline of some of the heartening research that is going on into the mechanisms and effect of homoeopathy. Note that the author is unable to support laboratory animal experimentation or any wilful causing of disease or suffering in animals. Such research is therefore not discussed.

1 Study of the homoeopathic potentised solutions to try to discover what principle is involved in their make-up. Why is a 'potentised' solution different from a simple diluted solution of the same concentration? Such work includes studies of the crystallisation properties of the solutions, viscosity studies, studies of the molecular structure of the solvent etc.

2 Clinical trials in doctors' and veterinary clinics to determine the efficacy of remedies against specific diagnosed syndromes in individual cases. Such studies include work on Hay Fever, Rheumatism, Travel Sickness, Feline Leukaemia (FeLV) etc.

3 Clinical trials in intensive farm situations to determine the efficacy of specific remedies in controlling specific problems e.g. Dystocia, Mastitis, Milk Fever etc. See Veterinary Record 1984 114 p. 216, Proceedings of LMHI Congress, Lyon 1985, International Journal for Veterinary Homoeopathy 1986 Vol. 1 No. 1 p. 15.

4 Clinical trials in boarding kennels and rescue kennels to ascertain the efficacy of the nosodes in the protection of dogs against the great epizootic diseases to which they are prone e.g. Kennel Cough (IJVH Vol. 2 No. 1 p. 45 with clarification addendum in Vol. 2 No. 2 p. 57), Distemper (IJVH Vol. 5 p. 8 1991), etc.

5 Provings on healthy human volunteers using potentised remedies. These studies are consistently providing evidence that remedies, in potency, can

produce an effect. Few have been performed on animals and the ethical implications of such work would be of concern.

6 Study of the electromagnetic and bioelectric effects of potentised solutions.

Such journals as the 'British Homoeopathic Journal', 'Homoeopathy Today', 'Homoeopathy', 'The Veterinary Record' and 'The Journal of The British Homoeopathic Research Group' serve to publish the results of British work in these fields. The International Journal for Veterinary Homoeopathy, founded in 1986, collected papers from all over the world on the subject of veterinary homoeopathy and research. This journal was subsequently taken over by 'Dynamis'.

It is only by continuing these efforts that the required proof of the efficacy of the homoeopathic method will be obtained and a better understanding of its mechanisms reached. When these objectives are realised, much more will be learnt about how to use homoeopathy because it should then be an accepted, widely used and widely discussed form of medicine with a healthy exchange of ideas bringing new lines of thought to everyone's notice. Roll on that day!

KENNEL COUGH TRIAL (summarised as an example)

At the time of an outbreak in a boarding kennel there were 40 dogs boarding. 37 of these contracted kennel cough in the initial infection. Of these, 18 had received kennel cough vaccine prior to admission, all 18 went down with the disease. Of the 22 non-vaccinated, 19 went down with it.

Nosodes were introduced to all new boarders as they arrived into the infected premises during November. 214 dogs were boarded in this period. Of these, 64 were vaccinated prior to entry. 3 of these went down with the disease. Of the 150 non-vaccinated, only 1 contracted the disease.

These results appear to show:

a) that kennel cough *nosode* is an effective preventive;
b) but conventional vaccination of dogs (mid-1980s) was not;
c) that vaccination appears to reduce the response to homoeopathy.

Uses of Homoeopathy in Conventional Medicine

It is interesting to note that the benefits of the homoeopathic mechanism are being exploited unwittingly by orthodox medicine in a great variety of ways, showing that with a small change in approach there are common areas between homoeopathy and conventional medicine. This is heartening for the future of medicine since it makes it all the more likely that an open mind to homoeopathy can be adopted. A few examples here will serve to illustrate the claim:

Digitalis: Toxic symptoms include prolonged systolic period and fibrillation. Uses for Digitalis (or its modern analogues) in conventional therapy include shortening systole and controlling fibrillation. This is a case of *similia similibus curentur*.

Sulphur: Many skin dressings contain sulphur to cure skin diseases. Symptoms of toxicity of sulphur, when applied topically, include skin irritation.

Arsenic: Arsenical compounds were used as an effective control of Swine Dysentery. Acute arsenic toxicity includes vomiting, watery diarrhoea often with blood, exhaustion, collapse and death. Chronic poisoning produces wasting and unthriftiness with a weak and irregular pulse. These are the symptoms of Swine Dysentery in acute and chronic form.

Copper: It is now widely accepted that copper bracelets (collars for dogs) can help some rheumatism/arthritis cases. It is arguable that those cases which do respond are homoeopathically indicated patients which would respond to copper in potency. (There may also be electrical field effects.)

Gold: Similar arguments could be applied for those patients who respond to gold injections.

Fluorine: This applies only to human medicine. Fluorine is administered to the population in some areas of the UK, via the drinking water, to prevent the symptoms of dental decay. Fluorine poisoning would produce exactly those symptoms! Sadly, a by-product of industry is used (Sodium Aluminium Fluoride) when Calcium Fluoride would be safer and more effective.

Quinine: Derivatives are still used to combat Malaria and this was the substance which Hahnemann 'proved' in his first studies in 1790 as capable of producing malaria-type symptoms.

Nux vomica: Nux has been used in modern times in *Stomach Powders* for cattle. It is used as a digestive aid and colic treatment. An upset digestion and abdominal pain are among the symptoms of *Nux vomica* poisoning.

Ipecacuanha: There is still a conventional proprietary compound cough remedy available which contains Ipecacuanha – a potent cough-producing substance!

Aspirin: It can be argued that aspirin works in a homoeopathic manner, producing joint pains if fed to healthy individuals. Conventional science has not yet fully explained its mode of action as a 'painkiller'.

Aesculus: Modern ointment for human haemorrhoids have been known to contain Aesculin, derived from the horse chestnut. Homoeopathically, Aesculus may be used to treat piles in humans.

APPENDIX 8

Acute Disease, Chronic Disease and the Miasms

It is beyond the scope of this book to go deeply into theories of Acute and Chronic disease and Hahnemann's Miasm theory but it is salutary to focus one's mind on the problem, even if only for a short while. Besides, one cannot read deeply into homoeopathic literature without coming across references to the Miasm theory of chronic disease. This discussion is put in the appendix since it is of philosophical and academic interest, rather than essential to the basic study of homoeopathy.

ACUTE DISEASE is of rapid onset and short duration and, if the attack on the body is not too severe, the basically healthy body will eventually throw off the disease and recover. If the onslaught is too severe then death will result.

CHRONIC DISEASE is one of long standing. The patient and the disease reach a type of equilibrium. There is no period of resolution.

Both words are sometimes erroneously used to imply a level of *severity of disease*. This is not implied in either word.

Hahnemann taught that one should, in the treatment of disease.

1 Select a homoeopathic remedy, that is, one which has the power to reproduce similar symptoms in a healthy body.
2 Try to resist suppressive antipathic treatment; this may produce, in the case of chronic disease, deeper, more difficult symptoms; and in the case of acute disease can convert it into a chronic disease.
3 Allow the remedy time to work. A chronic disease is deep seated and will not disappear immediately. Often, the order of cure follows the pattern:
   a) From within outwards (in the case of skin disease this can often involve a worsening of the skin condition before a cure is obtained).
   b) From centre to extremities.
   c) Newer symptoms disappear before older ones.

THE MIASM THEORY

Hahnemann believed that all chronic human diseases stemmed from three basic (infective) 'miasms': *Psora* (the itch), *Sycosis* (Gonorrhoea) and *Syphilis*. He believed that the many variations seen in chronic disease arise from the continued passage of these 'infections' through countless generations of humans and countless distinct individual constitutions, subjected to a great number of extrinsic factors. Suppression of the symptoms he believed led to a driving inward of the chronic disease so that it could express itself as Cancer, Asthma, Paralysis, Nervous Debility or Epilepsy (he cited many more examples). He believed that there is a dormant seat of one or other or any combination of the three miasms in most individuals and that this might flare up at any time, as a result of stress to the system, e.g.: puberty, marriage, childbirth, bereavement etc. Each of life's stresses can contribute to a breakdown of one's inherent resistance to the dominant miasm.

In modern times it is probably more constructive to speak of 'tendencies' rather than 'miasms'. The *Psora* corresponds to a tendency to deficient or incomplete reaction; the *Sycosis* to a tendency to an exuberant or excessive reaction; the *Syphilis* to a tendency to destructive (or self-destructive) pattern of reaction. There are those who prefer to cite Vaccinosis, Tuberculosis and Cancer as new 'miasms'. This author tends to classify them in terms of combinations of the original three, a concept that can be very helpful in the treatment of those conditions. These tendencies apply in animals too.

Hahnemann firmly believed that it was folly to study cellular processes and other detailed disease symptoms but that one should simply choose, for treatment, a homoeopathic remedy selected according to the similia principle. He said, in a similar vein, that it was folly to present the many and varied manifestations of chronic disease as separate diseases in themselves under a multitude of particular names or to try to adapt a certain general medicine to any of them.

A deeper study of his thoughts on this subject can be found in the Organon, see Appendix 5, but he implied hereditary and infective mechanisms.

Whether or not one can accept Hahnemann's archaic and definite views on chronic disease is open to question but if there is anything in what he said then modern views of chronic disease must change. His lack of modern scientific knowledge and his pedantic prose make his theories seem fanciful but one must resist the temptation to dismiss them out of hand. *Modern medicine still falls into the trap* of imposing certain general names on diseases as well as adapting certain general medicines to them. Those who intend to take up homoeopathy must, in order to derive the most benefit from the method, change their way of thinking from the latter and concentrate more on learning about a disease from its totality of symptoms rather than its name. A study of patterns of disease and disease tendencies in a body, classified according to Hahneman's three miasms or combinations of them can prove very useful in narrowing the choice of remedies for a given patient.

Always bear these points in mind when using Chapter 8 et seq. for guidance in choosing a remedy, the required remedy for a particular case may not be listed. Without this approach failure (always a possibility owing to our human frailty) is much more certain (see p. 52).

APPENDIX 9

Veterinary Surgeon's List of First Remedies Incorporating Home Starter List

Once having taken up the challenge of homoeopathy it is essential to have on hand a number of useful remedies for contingency purposes. I have made a list which I can recommend as being the ones most likely to be useful under most domestic circumstances. They also constitute a very useful list for the veterinary surgeon taking the first plunge. Without a handy list like this there is very little to guide one's choice from the several thousand remedies available. *It is of course, only the author's own opinion that includes certain remedies on this list and leaves out others.*

Internal Medicines
*Aconitum napellus
*Apis mellifica
  Argentum nitricum
*Arnica montana
*Arsenicum album
  Belladonna
*Bryonia alba
  Cantharis
  Caulophyllum
  Chamomilla
  Colocynthis
  Gelsemium
*Hepar sulph.
  Ledum
*Mercurius corrosivus
*Mercurius solubilis
  Petroleum

  Pulsatilla
*Rhus toxicodendron
*Ruta
  Sanicula
  Sepia
  Silica
  Symphytum
*Urtica

Lotions, ointments or creams
*Arnica
*Calendula
  Euphrasia Eye Lotion
  Hamamelis
*Hypericum

The particular uses of these remedies are given in Chapters 8–14 and one should refer to these chapters and further reading for a reasonable understanding of their need to go on an 'essentials' list. Some of the circumstances for using these remedies demand veterinary involvement to ensure that no medical trouble can ensue from failure to pick up important symptoms. For example an apparent cystitis in a cat, leading one to use *Cantharis* perhaps, could in fact be a case of urolithiasis in which the urethra is blocked and urination is obstructed. Veterinary examination will reveal this, owner treatment may not and delay could be fatal. Other remedies can be a useful adjunct to conventional veterinary methods, for example, *Arnica* and *Symphytum* in the case of a fractured leg. *Arnica* will reduce the tissue damage and bleeding and the resultant pain, *Symphytum* will hasten healing. Be assured that no harm can follow from the use of these remedies. There are no side effects but some repercussions can occur which can be mistaken for side effects.[†]

The common potencies obtainable are listed and explained in Appendix 3. The potencies used in this country are, by convention, different from those used in Europe and some of these are listed too.

---

* Signifies the remedies most useful in a home starter kit for animals.
† The one exception to the rule is the case of *Silica* which has the power to reawaken an old encapsulated lesion of tuberculosis. This is a very unlikely eventuality in this day and age. Care should also be taken if giving *Silica* to an animal which has a prosthesis. See also Provings p. 53, Recapitulation p. 51 and Aggravation p. 52.

Nutrition and Diet

It is of fundamental importance in good medicine to support the medical stimulus applied to the body (homoeopathic medicine) with optimal nutrition. Good feeding depends not just upon the supply of essential nutrients in correct proportions for an individual animal's needs for daily activity and metabolism along with renewal of tissues (the scientific side), but also upon the absence of unusable and potentially harmful substances (e.g. artificial colourings, flavourings and preservatives including manufactured anti-oxidants). The philosophy of good nutrition insists that not only are the above criteria followed but also that the nutrients should be supplied from the correct dietary ingredients, compatible with an animal's evolved biological and ethological needs (the philosophical side).

By and large, these objectives are best fulfilled, in the case of our dogs and cats, by the preparation of their diet by ourselves, at home, from fresh and wholesome (preferably organic to avoid agrochemicals) ingredients.

It is not within the scope of this small book to detail possible diets and their ingredients, this is best done in discussion with your homoeopathic veterinarian. Suffice it to emphasise here the integral importance of a good, natural diet which is formulated in a philosophically and scientifically sound way, away from the pressures of commercialism and profit.*

Water supply should also be of optimal quality with regard to impurities. Water can be filtered into a glass container or spring water can be purchased in glass bottles. Alternatively, a proprietary in-line filter can be fitted to the house's drinking water supply.

Food and water should be offered in china or stoneware receptacles and food should be minimally processed, using stainless steel, pottery or cast iron utensils. This importantly avoids the use of plastic, aluminium and 'non-stick' receptacles. Do not use a microwave oven.

* *Feeding Dogs the Natural Way*, Christopher Day, Chinham Publications

Nosodes

A nosode (from the Greek 'νοσος' – disease) is a homoeopathic remedy prepared from disease material. This may be diseased tissue, blood from a diseased patient, discharges from a diseased patient, secretions from a diseased patient or may even be prepared from pathogenic organisms. The term does not apply to remedies made from healthy tissues, discharges, secretions or free-living, non-pathogenic organisms. The required material is then subjected to the usual homoeopathic dilution and succussion process.

Nosodes fall into several categories, itemised for convenience:

1 **Nosodes with a homoeopathic proving**. Examples are *Tuberculinum, Psorinum, Medorrhinum, Lyssin*. These appear in Materia Medica books, just as do ordinary homoeopathic remedies, and can be used in accordance with their full symptom picture.

2 **Nosodes without a homoeopathic proving**. Such remedies are prepared from disease material and may be used to help cure or prevent the specific disease from which they were prepared. If they are used in the same animal from which the original material was taken, they may be called *autonosodes*. Examples are Mastitis nosode, Chlamydia nosode, Distemper nosode, Salmonella nosode etc. Examples of autonosodes are blood and urine autonosodes. **Isonosodes*** are nosodes prepared from a group of animals and used to treat that group or an individual within that group.

3 **Bowel nosodes**. These are nosodes researched by Paterson and others and recorded in the British Homoeopathic Journal 1950 Vol. XL No. 3. They are prepared from human faeces which has responded to different homoeopathic remedies. Each of the bowel nosodes is related either to a single homoeopathic remedy or a group of homoeopathic remedies (detailed in the reference

* N.B. author's own terminology.

given above). These nosodes are described in detail in the reference and may be used when one or other of their related remedies fail, in order to 'reopen' the case. They may even be used to start a case for which one of their related remedies may later prove helpful. This work applies to human medicine but has been used in pet animals with great success. However, there is room for work to identify 'animal bowel nosodes'.

Prevention of infectious diseases by nosodes is an increasingly widely practised form of prophylaxis, both in the single human and animal situation and in the herd, pack or colony situation. Trial work has been performed, demonstrating the potential for this practice (see Appendix 6).

However, medicolegally, there is some way to go before the practice is endorsed by the conventional medical and veterinary establishments. The work done to date is not sufficient to prove *beyond doubt* that the technique is a valid method of prevention of infectious diseases so claims made about efficacy should be guarded and treated with suspicion when read or heard. The author is careful not to confuse the technique with conventional vaccination, a practice with obvious parallels.

It is imperative that such materials are only obtained from very reliable sources and that the source of material is correctly identified, since otherwise there is no method of testing quality or relevance to any particular infectious disease situation. Some of the products for sale and currently marketed are prepared from orthodox vaccine products, rather than from the disease. The author is not certain of the validity or wisdom of this method.

Sadly, the use of nosodes for prevention is not yet recognised in the horse, dog or cat world by the bodies who make the rules for competition or those other animal-related activities which require conventional vaccination as a precondition of entry. Since these bodies require proof of efficacy, and the only acceptable method of proof appears to be animal experimentation, then there is apparently, for the time-being, an impasse.

When nosodes are to be used in the *treatment* of sick animals, suffering from the specific infectious diseases from which the nosodes are prepared, it is imperative to ensure that the animal is strong enough (the vital force sufficiently robust) to withstand the challenge by this almost isopathic stimulus. Should the animal's system be sufficiently under threat prior to treatment, the nosode could tip the balance the wrong way. For this reason, nosodes are mostly used in the safer, convalescent period of an infectious disease, in order to hasten the disease's departure and lessen the likelihood of relapse.

APPENDIX 12

Homoeopathy, Animals
and the Law

In the UK, the treatment of animals by any person other than a qualified veterinarian, is against the law. This is the result of legal efforts to protect animals. The major piece of legislation in this area is the Veterinary Surgeons Act 1966. The diagnosis, advice based upon the diagnosis or actual treatment of an animal is strictly confined to veterinarians. This makes life quite difficult for those who would seek homoeopathic help for their pets, since there are so few veterinarians using homoeopathy (although the number is increasing) and even fewer who have the homoeopathic qualification (VetMFHom).

In addition to this, those who seek help from a non-veterinarian may be liable under the 1911 Protection of Animals Act, if the subsequent treatments fail to alleviate suffering or even result in further suffering for the animal in question. Such practitioners do not even carry insurance for the treatment of animals.

The Medicines Act 1968 and subsequent provisions, including various EC Directives, states that only *licensed* medicines may be marketed carrying a medical claim. A medicinal product can only be licensed if it satisfies the criteria of the Ministry of Agriculture for safety, quality and efficacy. Many 'patent' homoeopathic and herbal products exist, and are vigorously marketed often by companies with questionable pedigrees, and which do not satisfy these criteria, yet have implied claims on the packaging. The buyer should beware of such marketing trends. The old phrase *'caveat emptor'* applies with full vigor.

The members of the BAHVS are not only qualified veterinary surgeons but are also guided by a Code of Practice which sets out clearly the correct steps to ethical delivery of veterinary homoeopathy. Those vets who, in addition, hold the Faculty qualifications in veterinary homoeopathy are further guided by the Faculty's codes.

Index

{221}

DOGS: HOMOEOPATHIC REMEDIES

George Macleod

Many dog owners today are looking for alternative ways to treat their pets when they fall ill. This book is for them. Written by a qualified veterinarian and world authority on the homoeopathic treatment of animals, this comprehensive guide introduces the key principles of homoeopathy and explains the nature of homoeopathic remedies. It includes advice on how remedies can be prepared and administered, as well as helpful information on healing the various canine bodily systems. There is practical guidance on canine viruses and bacterial diseases, including the diseases of puppyhood, making this book a must for any dog owner.

CATS: HOMOEOPATHIC REMEDIES

George Macleod

Many cat lovers today are looking for alternative ways to treat their pets when they fall ill. This book is for them. Written by a qualified veterinarian and world authority on the homoeopathic treatment of animals, this comprehensive guide introduces the key principles of homoeopathy and explains the nature of homoeopathic remedies. It includes advice on how remedies can be prepared and administered, as well as helpful information on healing the various feline bodily systems. There is also practical guidance on treating specific diseases and common feline ailments such as parasites, wounds and minor injuries.

CATS: HOMOEOPATHIC REMEDIES

George Macleod

Many cat lovers today are looking for alternative ways to treat their pets when they fall ill. This book is for them. Written by a qualified veterinarian and several authority on the homoeopathic treatment of animals, this comprehensive guide introduces the key principles of homoeopathy and explains the nature of homoeopathic remedies. It includes advice on how remedies can be prepared and administered, as well as helpful information on treating the various bodily systems. There is also practical guidance on treating specific diseases and common feline ailments such as parasites, wounds and minor injuries.

THE TREATMENT OF HORSES
BY HOMOEOPATHY

George Macleod

Today, many people interested in the welfare of horses turn to treatments such as homoeopathy when their animals fall ill. This book explains how homoeopathy offers a speedy and effective means to combat equine illness, often dealing with so-called 'incurable' ailments by the use of medicines that are absolutely safe, easy to administer and which have no side effects. Written by a qualified veterinarian and world authority on the homoeopathic treatment of animals, this comprehensive guide is the culmination of many years' experience in successfully treating horses. It introduces the key principles of homoeopathy and explains the nature of homoeopathic remedies. It includes advice on how remedies can be prepared and administered, as well as helpful information on healing a wide range of equine diseases and disorders.

Buy Rider Books

Order further Rider titles from your local bookshop, or have them delivered direct to your door by Bookpost

☐ **Dogs: Homoeopathic Remedies**
    by George Macleod   1844131963   £7.99
☐ **Cats: Homoeopathic Remedies**
    by George Macleod   1844131947   £7.99
☐ **The Treatment of Horses by Homoeopathy**
    by George Macleod   1844132951   £12.99

FREE POST AND PACKING
Overseas customers allow £2.00 per paperback

ORDER:
By phone: 01624 677237
By post: Random House Books
c/o Bookpost
PO Box 29
Douglas
Isle of Man, IM99 1BQ
By fax: 01624 670923
By email: bookshop@enterprise.net

Cheques (payable to Bookpost) and credit cards accepted

Prices and availability subject to change without notice.
Allow 28 days for delivery.
When placing your order, please state if you do not wish to receive
any additional information.

www.randomhouse.co.uk